WHY?

The Betrayal and Broken Promises to Our Children

BY
RAYMOND J. HEAD

WHY?
The Betrayal and Broken Promises to Our Children
By Raymond J. Head

To order more copies of this book in Paperback or Hardcover, or to receive information about other products, contact:
Nehas Publishing, LLC, 3227 Drummond Dr.
Stone Mountain, GA 30087,
or
www.rayjhead.com
ISBN: 9781456641504
Printed in the United States of America

About the Cover

First and foremost, I would like to thank the Book Marketing Pros for enhancing my vision, particularly the team who designed my book cover. The cover gives an endearing first impression, communicates what the book is about, and conveys the feeling you'll get from reading it. I humbly say (Asante sana) thank you all.

Moreover, the story behind the cover is equally intriguing. The image of me holding my twin daughters in that particular formation was captured over thirty years ago. I held them in a W formation as if I was asking Why me? As if I didn't already know.

My mother had five sets of twins and three before conceiving me. I was her first single birth which was said to be my blessing and my curse. In layman's terms, I would be the first of her children to have twins because I wasn't a twin.

Ase (It was so), our twin daughters Meghan and Rachel were born on October 24, 1992, making me the first of my mother's children to have twins. However, having twins was not a curse at all. It is a gift that keeps on giving. Little did we know, there was a reason we had our fraternal twin daughters. Both were born so that both could live.

Meghan was diagnosed with leukemia at seven months, exposing us to an insightful and intricate twenty-one-year journey. A journey where circumstances plotted our course, but wisdom, knowledge, and understanding completed our journey.

The day we received the lab results to determine the twins' bone marrow compatibility; was the day we understood how and why we were twice blessed with twins. The blood drawn from Rachel could have been Meghan's very own blood. Every aspect that could and should match for a compatible bone marrow transplant matched.

They were a match made in heaven. Without question, Rachel became Meghan's bone marrow donor. She did great. Rachel was walking about the day after the transplant with only two tiny pinholes, one on each hip, attesting to the lifesaving gift she gave her sister.

Twins Magazine, Special 12th Anniversary issue, July/August 1996, highlights Meghan's journey. Written by Tribune Head, entitled: A Match Made In Heaven. Meghan was a twenty-one-year cancer survivor. She transitioned on May 2, 2014.

I dedicated my first book, _From Plight to Promise_ to her. Meghan's strong desire to know the truth and her willingness to learn has given me the necessary motivation to tell the most extraordinary story ever, our story. The story that enthralled and informed her. Meghan is the ultimate reason I write.

I would be remiss if I didn't acknowledge my wife and soul-mate of thirty-two years. Together Tribune and I have weathered some of life's most difficult storms. We have also been the favored recipients of the joys and the fulfillments of this life.

Tribune's image is also on the cover, an image captured more than sixty years ago. She knew early on that she wanted to become a registered nurse. Tribune has served over forty years as a pediatric oncology nurse nurturing and caring for children with cancer.

Our Creator directed her path long ago, knowing it would take a special person to care for his children in the dreadful battle against cancer. When I think of models for developing human potentiality, Tribune is among those that come to mind.

On the cover are those with more time behind them than in front of them, those in their prime time, and those at the beginning of their time. More to the point, our children are the answer to the equation of the future, and knowledge is the common denominator.

Knowledge or the lack thereof will determine the haves and the have-nots. That being said, there is a dire need to provide the necessary cultural substance for all children, particularly children of color.

Educating our children is not an event; it is an essential process that will enable them to embrace the blueprint for obtaining an everlasting vision.

WHY?

In a nutshell, the cover speaks to and about the development of human potentiality and the reorientation of consciousness for our children. It projects love, respect, and passion. It reflects the variable and invariable nature of life and circumstances. It also taps into the themes of racism, oppression, and inequality and asks WHY?

Dedication

I dedicate this book to children of color and their parents globally, particularly Black American children. In the hope that it will serve as the necessary motivation to begin the vital process of restructuring the deeply structured inequalities we face as a people.

I thank God for all our children; they are indeed masters of destiny. Moreover, our Black children possess the innate ability to consciously contribute to the undoing of their fundamental and systemic challenges.

And I pray that this process will allow our children to embrace the reality that they are so much more than students of life; they are also profound teachers, and their lessons to come will be a new experience for the world to behold.

As the great Dr. Martin Luther King Jr. said, *"Our lives begin to end the day we become silent about things that matter." We will not stay silent, and we will not stop fighting- For our children's rights. His life informed us, and his dreams sustain us yet.*

Ase (It is so)

Preface

Sadly, true knowledge often gives way to distorted perceptions of reality, usually accepted as legitimate scholarship. Therefore, I will provide an unparalleled perception in Black and White.

As I begin writing while thinking about our children, their future, and the future of our nation, I'm reminded of the opening lines of the Declaration of Independence.

"We hold these truths to be self-evident that all men are created equal. Our creator has endowed us with certain unalienable rights, and among them are life, liberty, and the pursuit of happiness."

As my mind strolls down memory lane, I'm also reminded of the opening line of the Constitution and the final words of the Pledge of Allegiance:

"We, the people of the United States," and the last words of the Pledge of Allegiance are "liberty and justice for all."

Without question, the founding Fathers defined America clearly, with compelling words that cannot be misunderstood. These words placed America's citizens in a contract with one another to establish unity, tranquility, and justice to promote the general welfare of all.

These words also represent a sacred oath, committing ourselves to establish a society where all are free, treated with equal justice, and given equal opportunity to experience tranquility and happiness. These words are essential to our society, and if these words cease to have meaning, America will likely have an unfortunate and inescapable outcome.

Ironically, the insightful words of Frederick Douglass also come to mind. In his West India Emancipation speech on August 4, 1857, he stated with extreme certainty, *"If there is no struggle, there is no progress. Power concedes nothing without a demand. It never did, and it never will."*

These words are as insightful today as they were in 1857 due to the perpetuation of oppression through systemic racism. Let us be mindful that the existence of racism in America is not an opinion. It is a quantifiable fact, it was then, and it is now.

And to add insult to injury, the complex interactions of large-scale societal systems, practices, ideologies, and programs that produce and perpetuate inequities for racial minorities have become a societal norm.

My purpose for writing <u>Why?</u> is to expose, inform, and assist in restructuring the deeply structured inequalities we face as a people. While at the same time arming our children to address the primary concerns of Afrikan Americans henceforth.

My talking about racism is not an attempt to guilt or shame anyone. It is about spreading awareness so that it can be adequately addressed. Evoking change is a long process, but learning more about systemic racism is an essential first step.

As an Afrikan/American father, it is incumbent upon me to bring the truth to reality. I was humbled and honored that my daughters disciplined themselves and allowed me to be their teacher. Little did they know that for me to be their teacher, I had to first and foremost be an avid student, which has been highly empowering within itself.

More specifically, the added benefit is the humbling insight gained and the ability to share that insight in supporting, enhancing, and investing in our children, our people, and the future of our nation.

Ase (It is so)

Disclaimers

"Afrika" vs. "Africa"

As you will notice, I spell Afrika with a "K" instead of a "C" This is because most vernacular or traditional languages on the continent spell Afrika with a "K." Therefore, the use of "K" is relevant to us. We are confident the name spelled with the "C" came into use when Afrikan were dispersed worldwide. Therefore, the "K" symbolizes our coming back together again.

Using the letter "K" is my way of fulfilling my Ancestral Obligation regarding verifying and distributing factual knowledge and information. It's also a fundamental part of my activism in understanding and acknowledging the explicit nature of the word Afrika, spelled with a "K."

In the words of the Honorable Marcus Mosiah Garvey, in his outstanding work, *"Afrika for the Afrikans,"*

"In the spelling of Afrika, a "k" is used rather than a "c" because, for many activists, the "k" represents an acknowledgment that "Africa" is not the true name of that vast continent. When one speaks of Afrika, they bring an Afrikan- centered view of the meaning. Therefore, the Afrika spelled with a "k" represents a redefined and potentially different Afrika, it also symbolizes a coming back together of Afrikan people worldwide. Let it be understood that when one speaks of Afrika, and when most whites think of "Africa," they are coming from two different worldviews. One view supports the Afrikan ethos [spirit], while the other view supports the European ethos."

The Ancestors

The word 'Ancestors' is not a proper noun that requires capitalization. However, I adamantly choose to do so because the Ancestors are just that important in our Afrikan tradition and culture.

Black

The word "Black" is always capitalized in my book because it represents empowerment and challenges mainstream ideology.

Table of Contents

Introduction

Today's America is a fractured society, sharply divided by race, gender, religion, political party, and economic class. The roots of bias and unfairness still remain a perpetual part of America. More specifically, racism is so American that when we protest it, people think we are protesting America.

Because I embrace the belief that if we don't know who we are as a people, we won't know who we are as a person; therefore, it is incumbent upon me to reveal fundamental truths that are crucial for the survival of our people.

Equally important, our Black children must know and understand these life-altering truths. Moreover, most informed white Americans would agree that the influence of Black culture on America has been and will continue to be significant.

My initial intent is to inform my people, particularly our children, that we have a priceless heritage pleading for us to acknowledge and support. Mother Afrika instructs us to

1

"Know Thyself," and navigating through that process, I have confirmed that this knowledge resides in the womb of a rejected people and their way of life.

These irrefutable truths became even more apparent as I studied the pyramids, temples, and tombs while in Kemet (Egypt). At that point, Mother Afrika had convinced me that a legacy of money cannot replace a heritage of dignity.

Searching for and knowing our true identity is necessary because knowing eliminates the need to accept distorted, biased, created labels that do not reflect our true identity. Acknowledging our true identity as individuals or groups enhances life and liberty.

More specifically, identification is the first step in recognizing that our unique experience as a people, with its many triumphs and tragedies, is still the embodiment of totality representing who we truly are as Black people and children of a sovereign Creator.

Contrary to our current efforts, too many of our Black children are in crisis, caught in a twisted hip-hop culture, dropping out of school, ending up in jail, and having babies when they are not ready or even able to be parents.

Far too many of our youth have embraced today's stereotypical nonsense that has unfortunately passed as the new Black culture. And if not resisted and denounced, it will lead our children even further in a perilous direction.

<u>WHY?</u> Exposes and confronts the crimes of our nation and the broken promises that highlight the betrayal of our children. However, our nation's complicit behavior is not the only contributing factor to the betrayal of our children. Our complacent behavior and forgetfulness as their parents have also contributed to the overall betrayal of our children.

The late and distinguished Maya Angelou explains it best in her epic poem, <u>THE BLACK FAMILY PLEDGE.</u>

"BECAUSE we have forgotten our ancestors,

Our children no longer give us honor.

BECAUSE we have lost the path our ancestors cleared

Kneeling in perilous undergrowth,

Our children cannot find their way.

BECAUSE we have banished the God of our ancestors,

Our children cannot pray.

BECAUSE the old wails of our ancestors faded beyond our hearing,

Our children cannot hear us crying.

BECAUSE we have abandoned our wisdom of mothering and fathering,

Our befuddled children give birth to children, they neither want nor understand.

BECAUSE we have forgotten how to love, the adversary is within our Gates, and holds us up to the mirror of the world shouting, "Regard the Loveless"

Therefore, we pledge to bind ourselves to one another, to embrace our lowliest, to keep company with our loneliest, to educate our illiterate, to feed our starving, to clothe our ragged, to do all good things, knowing that we are more than keepers of our brothers and sisters. We ARE our brothers and sisters.

IN HONOR of those who toiled and implored God with golden tongues, and in gratitude to the same God who brought us out of hopeless desolation, we make this pledge."

I chose to begin with Maya Angelou's poem (The Black Family Pledge) because its content is central to the theme of WHY? It projects the ideology of universal brotherhood, love, and compassion but also taps into themes of hatred, ungratefulness, and forgetfulness.

More importantly, it highlights how black families have forgotten their past, how to love, and the cultural values that define them as a people, which have contributed to the betrayal and broken promises to our children.

However, a path to resolution is understanding that knowing ourselves is a fundamental aspect of assuming personal power and effectiveness, which is essential because the development of our children is based on the information they receive about themselves.

<u>WHY?</u> Exposes the devastating effects of the systemic challenges that our nation has created and perpetuated. Not only do these challenges negatively affect Black families presently, but they are designed to negatively affect our children for generations to come.

Through everything from banking to education, systemic racism has a smoother path to economic success for whites who exploit what Blacks have created.

<u>WHY?</u> Answers one of the most controversial questions of our time: Is "Critical Race Theory" a way of understanding how American racism has shaped public policy or a divisive discourse that pits people of color against white people?

<u>WHY?</u> Critiques the public education system in America, confronts racism, debates critical race theory, avidly engages in body talk, and reveals the need for preparing and healing our children. And last but not least, the question of Why is answered.

Ultimately, knowing who we are, where we come from, and where we still must go forces us to acknowledge that the system is not just broken but it was intentionally designed and built that way.

Therefore, we must understand that, as a people, it is not about the perfection of our walk; it is about the direction of our walk and "why."

Ase (It is so)

Chapter 1
Fundamental Understanding

Family is everything; it is the foundation of who we are. It is inherently designed to be suitable for children and adults. It includes all the descendants of a common Ancestor, and with that comes their history and values, such as love, respect, gratitude, and brotherhood. These values allow us to bind ourselves one to another, validating that we are more than just keepers of our brothers and sisters.

I have been a fan of Maya Angelou for decades, and I admire her work. She wrote and published _The Black Family Pledge_ in 2005, at a time when its message was needed and widely embraced. This poem resonated with me because of its ability to be powerful beyond measure.

The Breakdown

Not only does her inspiring revelation chastise us, but it also teaches and corrects us. She holds our nuances openly to the world by counting our faults one by one, providing a list of causes and effects concerning the attitude of Blacks in modern times.

Ultimately showing us that truth is a vital component of constructive criticism. The pledge also highlights the recommitting of values one should cherish to make this earth a desirable place to live and let live.

The pledge projects the ideology of universal brotherhood, love, and compassion, but it also taps into themes of hatred, ungratefulness, and forgetfulness. More importantly, it highlights how Black families have forgotten their past, how to love, and the cultural values which have affected our children.

I chose to write about our children because they are our future, and far too many of them are in crisis. When I ask myself why I am confronted with the harsh reality that we have yet to fulfill our obligation as Black parents.

As we have forgotten our past, our children follow the same path. They fail to honor our Ancestors who fought selflessly for their future generations. These are, in part, the irons that stoke the fires of ungratefulness within our children.

I chose to begin with Maya Angelou's poem because its content is central to the theme of Why?. Her masterful way of consciously opening a world of subliminal messaging is gripping. According to the poet, the adults have lost the path their Ancestors cleared.

The "path" is a metaphor for the advancement of the community, and the problems faced are referred to as the "perilous undergrowth," alluding to slavery, inequality, broken promises, and betrayal.

She states that as we have already lost track, our children are confused and wandering without knowing which way to go. Therefore, we must show them who they are and where they come from; this vital process will aid them in determining which way to go.

Unwisely, we have banished the God of our Ancestors, resulting in the deviation and loss of our spiritual and religious values. I believe that one of the reasons Black people continue to suffer spiritually is because they still worship the God assigned to them by their former enslavers.

Further, descendants of the same people with the same mentality still actively encourage many of us to worship European images and concepts that have caused us to become the principal agents in our spiritual destruction and confusion. Therefore, our children have also lost faith in the divine power, and they hunger spiritually.

This is crucial to understand because religion and spirituality are resting places for one's culture and are primary factors in shaping the way most perceive life in their world of reality. And it is often a determining factor in the outcome of one's plight.

In a later stanza, Maya Angelou talks about the "old wails" of our Ancestors, alluding to the suffering of those who fought for the emancipation of the community from the shackles of slavery, inequality and subjugation. Thus leaving scars of emotional detachment reflected in our children, not allowing them to hear us crying.

Abandoning the wisdom of parenting speaks to our babies having babies that they are unable or unwilling to parent. Have we forgotten that to get love and respect, we must show the same to our children?

We must ask ourselves, have we truly forgotten how to love, and if so, why? The poet holds us up to the mirror of the world and shouts, "Regard the loveless," labeling us as the hearts that have forgotten how to love.

After uttering this necessary list of cause and effect, she presents a road map to guide us in reaching our maximum potential by sowing seeds that benefit others.

The pledge is to bind one to another, filling the gaps by holding each other's hands like a human chain. And because a chain is only as strong as its weakest link, we pledge to embrace, enhance, and reinforce.

Maya also advocates for the lowliest, the loneliest, the illiterate, the hungry, and the ragged while subliminally highlighting the ideas of education for all and the eradication of hunger and poverty.

Pledging to do all good things, knowing that we are more than keepers of our brothers and sisters. WE ARE our brothers and sisters. This passage highlights the precepts and practices of universal brotherhood and human dignity.

In the last stanza, the poet indicates that this pledge is taken in honor of those who toiled and implored God with their "golden tongues," symbolizing our Ancestors' powerful and valuable voices. Therefore, we must be grateful to our Ancestors as well as to God, who brought them out of their "hopeless desolation."

For that reason, the present generation is reaping the fruits of their Ancestors' labor that have provided a path to freedom, opportunity, and education. _The Black Family Pledge_ highlights several reasons Black families are now facing multiple challenges. In part, the present generation with their lack of gratitude, is struggling due to their parents' forgetfulness of their past.

It is essential that the present generation understand that fundamental challenges can be addressed with fundamental understanding. Moreover, we Black parents must understand and teach our children that to know where we're going, it is imperative to know where we've come from.

Understanding this principle is crucial because we can interpret our present and project our future when we know our past. This understanding is also the start of a vital process designed to build value, shape character, and establish accountability within our children for— future generations.

Fundamental Understanding Brings Fundamental Change

It has been said, "Nothing succeeds like success," and that has a lot of truth to it. Let us be mindful that our Afrikan traditional culture, heritage, and history is the longest-running success story ever. Equally important, if we did it before, we can and must do it again.

As a people, we must realize that the study of Afrika is essential. Without her, we can't know our history or heritage; without that knowledge, we can't know ourselves or sufficiently aid our children in establishing who they are, where they come from, and where they still must go

In her outstanding work *"In the Spirit,"* Susan Taylor states with extreme certainty, "If this world had a righteous plan for you and me, we would have been taught early on how to give love to ourselves in a real way...How to delight in our collective history...But the world doesn't offer that- particularly to Black folk. We must struggle and invent to learn it on our own."

Our children are often put in adverse situations due to a lack of knowledge, primarily by systematic design. However, we now have the knowledge and the necessary motivation to correct these systemic challenges. In doing so, we must understand that our children learn what they live and often live what they learn.

As I'm writing and sipping tea in my favorite cup, I begin to reminisce on some of my personal experiences regarding children that have profoundly affected how I view our children and our future.

Almost thirty years ago, a good friend gave me this cup, knowing I was about to embark on the challenge of single parenting with a young daughter. I didn't know then, but I know now that she gave me more than just a cup.

I never thought a cup could teach me so much, but it did. I now understand that a child's God-given nature and innocence show us who we truly are.

Children Learn What They Live

Around the top and the bottom of the cup are children of all nationalities holding hands, forming a human chain, and it reads,

Children Learn What They Live
If a child lives with criticism-He learns to condemn.
If a child lives with hostility-He learns to fight.
If a child lives with ridicule-He learns to be shy.
If a child lives with shame-He learns to feel guilty.
If a child lives with tolerance-He learns to be patient.
If a child lives with encouragement- He learns confidence.
If a child lives with praise- He learns to appreciate.
If a child lives with fairness- He learns justice.
If a child lives with security-He learns to have faith.
If a child lives with approval-He learns to like himself.
If a child lives with acceptance and friendship-He learns to find love in the world.

This poem illustrates a cause-and-effect relationship that shows us how children develop. Dorothy Law Nolte wrote and first published this inspirational poem in 1954.

Still, long before that, The Bible speaks of our children in leadership roles, helping bring about balance and harmony, peace and tranquility. Isaiah 11:6 is an excellent illustration; it tells us:

"The wolf will live with the lamb, the leopard will lie down with the goat, the calf and the lion and the yearling together, and a little child will lead them."

Isaiah speaks of a time yet to come, a time of peace when children can play with formerly dangerous animals. In understanding the imagery of Isaiah's time, the dangerous animals spoken of are metaphors for predatory nations and oppressive systems that will no longer hurt or destroy God's children.

He also states that a little child will lead them; whether Isaiah meant that figuratively or not, it brings us back to a child free of oppression. This time is still yet to come for people of color, particularly children of color.

Today's systemic challenges consist of complex interactions of large-scale societal systems, practices, ideologies, and programs that produce and perpetuate inequities for racial minorities, intentionally designed and implemented to hinder our children's ability to lead.

These elements are indicative of the same predatory and oppressive systemic challenges that Isaiah spoke of. Think about this, if there are no children with the ability to lead there is no future for the people they represent. That's what the powers that be (the system) count on. Therefore, we must change that by seeing beyond our own time.

The Masters of Destiny

My soulmate comes to mind as I continue to write and ponder on the children. Tribune has worked as a pediatric oncology nurse for forty-one years, and she is truly a special person. I believe our Creator directed her path long ago, knowing it would take a special person to care for his children in the battle against cancer.

I'm often pleasantly reminded of our first real conversation getting to know one another. We talked for over two hours. I explained that I was a single dad with a young daughter, and we had to be a package deal.

To make a long story shorter, Tribune agreed to go out with me and requested that I meet her children at some point. This revelation threw me for a loop because we had talked for over two hours, and she never mentioned that she had children.

However, she was referring to her children at the hospital where she worked, and meeting her children has given me a whole new perspective on children in general. I had no idea that there were so many children affected by cancer.

Unfortunately, about two years into our marriage, cancer reared its ugly head in our lives, affecting our twin daughter Meghan. She was diagnosed with leukemia at seven months, exposing us to an insightful and intricate twenty-one year journey that showed us the variable and invariable nature of life and circumstances.

It gave us the necessary wisdom, knowledge, and understanding to address life's uninvited issues. We truly learned to embrace the concept that nothing that comes stays, and nothing that goes is lost.

Meghan was without question one of the most inspirational catalysts with respect to my spiritual walk and overall growth from her sunrise to her sunsetting. Not only did she bring about a heightened level of spiritual consciousness, but she also brought with her a set of circumstances that started us on an intricate and insightful journey.

A journey where circumstances plotted our course, but wisdom, knowledge, and understanding completed our journey. Meghan's journey showed us that as children of a sovereign Creator, we are never victims of our circumstances. Meghan is the ultimate reason I write.

Tribune's young patients are from all walks of life, and they all have one common denominator. They are in a battle against cancer. These amazing children taught me how to embrace life as it presents itself. Ultimately enabling me to find comfort in the face of adversity.

More specifically, the resiliency of these children amidst this dreadful battle against cancer is phenomenal and unmatched. It is evident that they are both profound students and teachers of life, reflecting who they truly are and who we were truly meant to be.

Our children are the masters of destiny, and it's worth our time and effort to assist them in getting where they must still go.

Destiny and the Dream

The dream I'm referring to is the so-called ever-changing American Dream or for some, The American Nightmare. The American Dream has been exalted to the point that it makes it something it was never meant to be. Further, It has resulted in a disappointing ideology for people of color

The American Dream should not be a one-size-fits-all concept, particularly when most can't reach it. It should be an unbiased, fluid notion that embodies the principles of the U.S. Constitution in practical philosophy. Understanding that those practicalities change with every generation.

The American Dream should be a dream of social order in which each man and each woman shall be able to attain the fullest stature of which they are innately capable. And be recognized by others for what they are, regardless of the fortuitous circumstances of birth or position.

With that being said, I'm reminded of my volunteer work and time spent with the children at "YES! Atlanta" as a committed partner for their Rising Star Vll program dealing with at-risk youth. It was indeed a humbling learning experience.

The youth were considered Millennials and Generation Z, and their dream priorities differed significantly from mine. As a baby boomer, my dream priorities were financial independence, home ownership, and providing an unshakable foundation for my children.

The phrase "American Dream" was first made famous by the historian James Truslow Adams in his 1931 book _The Epic of America._ There has also been the American Dream of a land where life should be better, richer, and fuller for every man, with opportunity for each according to his ability or achievement.

Ironically, it is a difficult dream for many Europeans to interpret adequately: too many of us have grown weary and mistrustful of it. Each generation must customize the American dream to fit its own circumstances and realities at that time. Therefore, we must encourage the members of Generation Z and beyond to prioritize their own values.

Many say Generation Z is technically the future, but it's a default setting, not a spiritual calling. I say it's destiny. Destiny is the events that will necessarily happen to a particular person, group of people, or thing in the future. It embodies the hidden power believed to control what will happen in the future. Fate is that hidden power in the development of events beyond one's control. Its regarded as determined by a supernatural power/force.

More to the point, most of us agree that one part of the American dream that cannot be changed or compromised is the commitment to make the opportunity for a better, more prosperous, and fuller life available to everyone.

Knowing

Every child's path to adulthood—reaching developmental and emotional milestones, learning healthy social skills, and dealing with problems is different and challenging.

Unfortunately, there is no map, and the road is never straight.

More specifically, children of color, particularly Black children, face added challenges along the way that are often beyond their control, accompanied by the challenges that today's generation of young people face are unprecedented and uniquely difficult to navigate.

However, knowing ourselves is a fundamental aspect of assuming personal power and effectiveness, which is essential because the development of our children is based on the information they receive about themselves.

Equally important, we as a people must dispel the accepted myths that the Western world and history have perpetuated for centuries regarding Black people, particularly in American history, where the history of Black people starts at the point of slavery.

After that, we are portrayed as insolvent debtors and regarded as an underclass of people representing the perpetuation of an oppressive cycle that has negatively affected Black people for generations. And to add insult to injury, this process did not happen accidentally.

Therefore, the earlier we start our indoctrination process to counter the devastating systemic attacks on our children, the earlier we begin arming them for generations to come. As Afrikan American/Black people, it is crucial that we look beyond and rise above the image of Afrika and her descendants created for us and the entire world by Europeans.

As Afrikan people, have a cultural memory that extends deep enough to recapture the cultural wealth that has given us the potential that has made us a great people. There are various levels and stages of socialization, but first and foremost, we must aid our children in establishing who they are, where they come from, and where they still must go.

This necessary process will enable our children to avidly embrace their cultural wealth by inherently understanding that their culture was initially designed to give meaning to reality.

If we seize this moment for our children and their families in their time of need and lead with inclusion, kindness, and respect, we can lay the foundation for an even healthier, more resilient, and much more fulfilled nation.

Ultimately, ensuring healthy children and families will take a societal effort, including policy, institutional and individual changes in how we view people of color, particularly Black people.

Ase (It is so)

Chapter 2

Who We Are, Where We Come From, and Where We Still Must Go

Why it's Important

Kareem Abdul-Jabbar and Raymond Obstfeld, in their outstanding work _Writings On The Wall/Searching For A New Equality Beyond Black And White,_ explain why history is so important:

"History illuminates the safest path in front of us by revealing the pitfalls of the past. It is a secular bible of cautionary and inspiring stories that distills the wisdom of thousands of years of human endeavors into practical lessons about humanity's morals, politics, and personal relationships. It is the ultimate self-help book.

However, in the hands of the greedy, the power-hungry, and the unscrupulous history is also a powerful tool of mass manipulation. It can be used to herd the unaware into self-destructive choices."

Without question, history is open to interpretation. However, it is crucial for children of color, particularly Black children, to understand that history can be a critical guide to their present and future, both personally and culturally. However, the consequences of being unaware of our history can be devastating.

Therefore, it is necessary to search for and know our true identity. Knowing will eliminate the need to accept distorted, biased, created labels that do not reflect who we truly are. Knowing our true identity is also fundamental in assuming personal power and effectiveness.

Identity is the first step in recognizing that our unique experience, with its many triumphs and tragedies, still embodies totality, representing who we truly are as Black people and children of a sovereign Creator.

Despite the issues of race, racism, and sexism, there is only one race, "the human race," which has been irrefutably proven to have originated in Afrika. And only those who have been successfully mis-educated have no desire to know their past and often resent those who do.

On My Journey

As you all know, I'm a baby boomer who grew up in the 60s and 70s and has seen some turbulent times in America, particularly for Black Americans. As I write about and to our children, I begin reminiscing about my childhood and some of the things that influenced me.

First and foremost, I am genuinely grateful for my village and all of those who served as fundamental cornerstones in making it all possible. Throughout this book, I will continue referencing the need to instill in our children a respect for education and an understanding of the power associated with attaining knowledge because it is a necessary tool. It was then, and it is now.

Then was February 1969 Negro History Week; I was eleven and in the sixth grade. Mr. Stewart was my teacher and, without question, an essential cornerstone of our village. He persuaded me to recite Dr. Martin Luther King Jr.'s; *I Have A Dream* speech as a part of our Negro History Week program. My experience was definitely perspective-altering, bringing truth to my reality.

I was taught from an early age that whatever I decided to do, I had an obligation to do my best. I wanted to do more than just recite the speech. I tried to deliver it with feeling and emotion because it was perhaps Dr. King's most well-known and most quoted address.

My father suggested that I go through the speech line by line and focus on what's being said and how I feel about it. He advised me to be objective and subjective while being opened minded all at the same time. And that I did.

I Have a Dream was Dr. King's keynote address of the March on Washington, D.C., for Civil Rights and a plea for justice and freedom. He delivered this speech before the Lincoln Memorial on August 28, 1963.

My delivery was excellent; I received an overwhelming standing ovation, but even more importantly, after understanding the content and purpose of this speech, my view of the world and how I saw myself in it changed dramatically.

Even though my delivery took place in our school auditorium, I felt as if I was at the Lincoln Memorial. Ultimately, understanding the theoretical and practical aspects of the speech put me there.

Dr. King's, *I Have A Dream* speech was, in a sense, our (the Negro People) coming to the nation's capital to cash a check. Dr. King exclaims:

"When the architects of our republic wrote the magnificent words of the Constitution and the Declaration of Independence, they were signing a promissory note to which every American was to fall heir. This note was the promise that all men, yes Black men as well as white men, would be guaranteed the unalienable rights of life, liberty, and the pursuit of happiness.

It is obvious today that America has defaulted on this promissory note in so far as her citizens of color are concerned. Instead of honoring this sacred obligation, America has given the Negro people a bad check, which has come back marked "insufficient fund." We refuse to believe that there are insufficient funds In this great nation's vaults of opportunity.

And so we've come to cash this check, which will give us upon demand the riches of freedom and the security of justice."

This experience was indeed a crucial turning point for me. More specifically, it furthered my desire to know who I am, where I come from, and where I still must go. Ultimately, I came to the realization that Black History is a 24/7, 365-day-a-year occupation assigned to me by the Creator himself.

What I Have Learned

I can say with certainty that the story of the Afrikan Legacy is the most incredible story I have ever told. First and foremost, Afrika is the home of humanity, producing a people of first, setting the genesis for all future civilizations. Think about that!

I now understand and acknowledge that the foundation of the belief system of the world today was birthed, established, and implemented first on the immense continent of Afrika.

Afrika is collectively known as the "Motherland," and rightfully so, because within her lies the fallopian tube of civilization, representing life itself, thereby making her the parent of all past, present, and future civilization.

Equally important, Black history should be important to everyone, not only because it's the history of Black people, but because it is the history of a people who have had a profound impact on world civilization. Our story is indelible because it tells of humanity's earliest events or actions. Our Ancestors irrefutably put the first footprints on the sands of time; that's a mouthful.

Our Experience Then and Now

Then

Let's face it; there are some things we can color-coat and others we can't. Unfortunately, the Black experience in America cannot be color-coated. It's in Black and White.

In his remarkable book, _They Stole It, But You Must Return It,_ Dr. Richard Williams takes a unique but appropriate approach to examining the historical aspect of the Black family. "They" refers to White America, and "You" refers to Black America.

He starts the book by explaining that usually, the thief must take responsibility and pay equal value for what he stole. However, with White America, this did not happen. They stole it, but you must return it.

The term White America refers to a specific group of Caucasians living in America. Not all Caucasians are in this group. White America refers to the white Caucasian segment of America that advocates racial hatred and promotes social injustices. That part of America violates the American creed of freedom and justice for all.

The term Black America, as used in his book, refers to all Afrikan/Americans- those in the United States, Canada, the Caribbean, South America, Europe, and other countries. It also refers to our brothers and sisters in Afrika. They, too, have been affected by the European countries in much the same way Afrikan/Americans have been affected by the United States and England.

To understand the problems of the Black family today, you must understand the experience and circumstances under which these problems developed. To create an effective slave system, White America focused on destroying the positive self-image of Blacks and their entire family structure.

After being snatched and stolen from his homeland and family, the Afrikan experienced a tragic trip across the Atlantic Ocean. This water route to America was called the Middle Passage. This trip set a trend of horrific experiences that would affect his descendants for generations.

Let us also be mindful that Afrikans were the only immigrants who came to America against their will, and the enslavement of Afrikans by non-Afrikans was based solely on race and greed.

Dr. Williams stated with extreme certainty that, *"Any system that deprives a people of its family structure denies the humanity of that people. The developers of such a system defy the Creator of mankind and insult the Creator's creation. White America originated such a system in its slavery scheme. White America introduced a new and different type of slavery. It was designed to destroy all elements of the Black family. History has no equal to match the terrible way in which White America treated and destroyed the Black family. White America stole it, but Black America must return it."*

White America attacked the dignity of the fathers, the mothers, and the children of the Black family in an attempt to eliminate the family concept by destroying the dignity of its components.

To understand the mentality of White America and its slavery scheme, we must have a clear understanding of what we are truly dealing with.

Ephesians 6:12 For we wrestle not against flesh blood, but against principalities, against powers, against the rulers of the darkness of this world, against spiritual wickedness in high places.

Now

There has been deliberate destruction of Afrikan culture and the records relating to that culture, starting with the first invaders of Africa. It continued through the period of slavery and the colonial system and continues today on a much higher and even more devastating level.

Although physical slavery has ended in the United States, its counterpart, mental slavery, continues to this day. Mental slavery affects the mind and can be just as bad or worse than physical slavery. Mental bondage is invisible violence with a self-containing mechanism.

What this means for those in bondage is not only will they fail to challenge beliefs and patterns of thought which control them, they will defend and protect those beliefs and patterns of thought.

Suppose our children grow up believing that the child who stares back at them in the mirror is inferior and incapable of correct thoughts or actions. In that case, they will become mentally enslaved to thoughts of inferiority.

Imprisonment is the new slavery for the Black community. On average, states spend over three times as much per prisoner compared to each public school student. Unfortunately, Black children are disproportionately denied a fair chance, often resulting in an unleveled playing field from birth.

This has contributed to many poor Black children getting pulled into a cradle-to-prison-to-death cycle that we must stop if the clock of racial and social progress is not to turn backward. Ultimately, the perceptions of reality that you have in your mind will either free you or keep you enslaved.

I don't have all the answers, but I know with certainty that developing and implementing new strategies is vital to ensure our survival. To free our children from mental bondage, we must have a strategy that includes mental, physical, and cultural nurturing.

Therefore, parents who are ignorant of their history and culture and have a total disregard for change will be incapable of adequately directing the lives of their children.

Who We Are

We are the product of the greatest creators and survivors on planet Earth. However, the survival experience has left some long-lasting consequences that affect Black Americans today.

We have been kings and queens, common folk, and enslaved people. I'm often asked how does the fact that we were kings and queens in Afrika help me survive today and how does this knowledge help me get a job and put food on the table?

First and foremost, we must understand the power associated with attaining knowledge. We must also understand that the key to successfully navigating our circumstances lies in knowing who we are, tapping into that Ancestral and cultural reservoir, and applying that knowledge.

One of the most significant and engaging facts regarding the kings and queens of the Afrikan Dynasties is that they served as models for the development of human potentiality then and now.

Let us also note that only a tiny percentage of the population in Afrika were kings and queens and members of the holy royal family. Most of the populous in any kingdom were ordinary folk, farmers, carpenters, healers, and the like.

They developed their individual skills, formed trade associations, and offered their services to the community. These are the people responsible for some of the most powerful expressions of human creativity.

Afrika instructs us to know thyself; this knowledge resides in the womb of a rejected people and their way of life. The real problem is that most of us don't realize that we are the rejected people who have surrendered our name and culture, which was an integral part of our initial way of life.

Losing our name and culture has resulted in our loss of appetite. Even when those among us recreate our culture and present it to us, we no longer have an appetite for it.

We have a greater desire for the culture of people other than ourselves.

No nation in the history of civilization has had a more significant influence on the arts and sciences than our homeland. The civilization of Afrika is the first civilization recorded in history having over three thousand years of cultural and historical continuance. That is a privilege that no other nation or people on this planet have experienced.

The same wisdom, knowledge, and insight our Ancestors had yesterday we have today. If appropriately utilized, it will not only get you a job; it will allow you to create jobs and abundantly put food on your tables. Equally important, we must never forget that power comes in knowing.

Where We Come From

We come from a place of cultural and historical wealth that serves as a model for the development of human potentiality. Therefore, it is imperative to know where we come from in order to know where we're going.

I am a Black man with a distinctive past. I am of Afrikan descent, as we all are to some degree or another. More importantly, I can accept or admit the existence or truth of that irrefutable fact.

From Egypt, my journey took me south to Ethiopia, an ancient country located in the Horn of Afrika. Anthropologists acknowledge Ethiopia as the place where humans originated.

It is an ancient land establishing one of the oldest civilizations in the world, if not the oldest.

The oldest fossil remains of a 3.18-million-year-old hominid known as Dinknesh was found in eastern Ethiopia in 1974.

She was called "Lucy" by the excavators who located her, but her Ethiopian name is Dinknesh, which means "thou are wonderful." She stood just under four feet tall and was an Ancestor of the modern hominid who walked upright.

In 1997, a fossilized skull of Idaltu was discovered in the Afar region of eastern Ethiopia. It was dated 160,000 years ago, making his fossil the earliest of modern humans or homo sapiens. The name Idaltu comes from the Afar word "firstborn."

These are essential factors in the chronology of Ethiopian history. More to the point, they are fundamental in the documentation and verification of why and how the Afrikan continent is the home of humanity and the parent (Mother) of all civilization.

No matter how we look at it or choose to see it, all relevant roads and avenues of approach lead us back to the original source; Mother Afrika, the home of humanity and a people of firsts.

Knowing where we come from will also help dispel some of the accepted myths that the Western world and history have perpetuated for centuries regarding Black people.

Where We Still Must Go

We still must go to a place of radical reorientation of our consciousness, but first and foremost, we must understand that in order to know where we're going, it is imperative to know where we've come from.

Further, until we wrestle with the demons that have shaped and framed us, we will not be able to embrace the full measure of our true humanity as citizens in society.

Understanding that "There Is No Future for a People Who Deny Their Past." forces us to realize that we have a cultural memory that extends deep enough to recapture the cultural wealth that has given us the potential that has made us a great people.

There are many elements in getting where we still must go, but knowing who we are and where we come from are the fundamental cornerstones upon which we must begin our building.

The truthful knowledge of Afrikan history and its application will serve as a crucial step toward the continued liberation of Afrikan people for generations to come. Let us also be mindful that all history is a current event. Therefore, nothing that comes stays, and nothing that goes is lost.

The Haves and the Have Nots

Mother Afrika has thoroughly convinced me that a legacy of money cannot replace a heritage of dignity. Mother Afrika also instructs us to "Know Thyself," in doing so, I have found that this knowledge resides in the womb of a rejected people and their way of life.

Knowledge is crucial because power comes in knowing. Knowledge is also essential in developing a sound belief system, one that is based on facts, truth, evidence, and justified belief. Without question, for us to move forward purposefully as a people, we must have the knowledge of what happened to our Ancestors in the past.

Moreover, this knowledge will allow us to find our way out of the mental and spiritual confusion most of us have been taught to accept uncritically. Despite the profound disdain history has shown for our people and our story, it only solidified that education begins at home. It always has and always will.

Initially, as a Black father, I told my children our story to bring truth to their reality and to build character by showing and teaching them the distinctive nature of our Afrikan origin.

Ultimately, our story was to provide education for transformation by acknowledging the established precedents of our spiritual, historical, and cultural significance as Black people.

I can not stress enough; parents and elders take the time to instill within our children a respect for education and an understanding of the power associated with the attainment of knowledge. And let us not forget that an education is not only an investment in the child's future; it's an investment in the entire family.

More importantly, we as parents and elders must engage our children even more with our story because it will provide the ultimate cultural substance necessary to obtain an everlasting vision. Our story will also give us, the parents and elders, the method and means to provide the crucial blueprint for that vision.

Carter G. Woodson, in his outstanding work *The Mis-Education of the Negro,* reminds us that:

"Philosophers have long conceded...that every man has two educations: that which is given to him, and the other that which he gives himself. Of the two kinds the latter is by far the more desirable. Indeed all that is most worthy in man he must work out and conquer for himself. It is that which constitutes our real and best nourishment. What we are merely taught seldom nourishes the mind like that which we teach ourselves."

Our innate knowledge and its application will aid us in knowing what must be done to enhance our future. However, knowing our history is vital because when we know our past, we can interpret our present and project our future.

It has been said that those who cannot remember the past are condemned to repeat it. Yet, society justifies its past mistakes by conveniently forgetting them or rewriting history. Ultimately, "Knowledge" or the lack thereof will determine "The Haves and the Have Nots."

A note to Black America: *"You are truly a miracle, and your future can be bright because you possess an inner strength and sensitivity that is unmatched. Once this power is aggressively and productively released, Black Americans and the Whole World will have a new experience."*

Hotep (Peace)

Chapter 3
Our Youth / Black Children

This chapter taps into the theme of betrayal and broken promises to our youth, notably children of color, who have no power to defend themselves. It exposes and confronts the crimes of our nation regarding public education in America and offers a fundamental ideology for a resolution.

Education System

Public education is facing a crisis unlike anything in decades, and it reaches into almost everything educators do, causing unprecedented stress levels in their daily lives. Today, the cascading problems are felt acutely by administrators, teachers, and students who walk the halls of our public schools across our country.

At the start of the pandemic, experts predicted that students forced into remote schooling would pay an academic price, and they were right. The toll of illness, death, and disruptions to a dependable routine and remote learning have left students academically behind, particularly children of color and those from low-income families.

The numbers are all going in the wrong direction for public schools. Enrollment is down, absenteeism is up, and there aren't enough teachers or substitutes, and each phase of the pandemic aftermath brings new logistics to manage.

Many teachers and students say they are emotionally drained, and experts predict schools will struggle with the fallout for years to come. Further, developing a plan to take schools in the right direction is easier said than done. The first challenge lies in identifying underlying problems that keep students from learning.

This challenge, in part, is because the problems may change considerably depending on who's labeling them, whether its students, parents, educators, or lawmakers. Let us briefly consider some significant challenges facing public schools based on the perspective of many in the world of education.

1. Classroom Size: Classroom numbers are often impacted when money gets tight. Yet, most teachers agree that they cannot effectively teach every student in a classroom if the class size exceeds the maximum limits.

2. Poverty: A report from the Southern Education Foundation, which shows in 17 states across the U.S., cites that low-income students now comprise the majority of public school students in those states

3. <u>Family Factors</u>: Family factors affects teacher's ability to teach students, what happens at home will impact a student's learning propensity.

4. <u>Technology</u>: Technology must come into the classroom to keep up with the learning demands of the 21st century.

5. <u>Bullying</u>: Bullying is not a new problem, but it has a profound impact on the learning aptitude of many students. Cyberbullying has also become a significant issue.

6. <u>Student's Attitudes and Behaviors:</u> Many public school teachers cite student attitudes, such as apathy and disrespect for teachers, as a significant problem facing schools today.

7. <u>No Child Left Behind</u>: Countless students, parents, and teachers see No Child Left Behind as a detriment to the public education environment. Its focus in education on the national and state level continues to be on the testing process.

8. <u>Parent Involvement</u>: Parental involvement is one of the most significant contributions to students' academic success, but teachers don't always get adequate participation from parents.

9. <u>Student Health:</u> Obesity has reached epidemic proportions in the U.S., and poor eating habits that lead to obesity problems may also contribute to low student achievement.

10. <u>Funding</u>: Budget cuts have created enormous problems for most public schools. Less funding means smaller staff, fewer resources, and a lower number of services for students.

There are numerous problems in public schools today, but identifying those issues is half the battle. More importantly, with a grocery list of challenges to face, now is the time for educators, parents, and lawmakers to come together and find solutions for the benefit of all students in public schools.

Eye Opening

About fifteen years ago, while researching South Afrika's apartheid era, I came across Jonathan Kozol's bestseller, <u>The Shame of the Nation–The Restoration of Apartheid Schooling in America.</u> It was indeed an eye-opener.

His book is a triumph of firsthand reporting, paying tribute to those educators who persist against the odds but directly challenge the chilling practices forced upon our urban systems by the Bush administration.

Kozol reported on the nearly sixty schools he visited over several years, virtually everywhere. He found that conditions had worsened for inner-city children since federal courts began dismantling the landmark ruling in Brown v. Board of Education.

He also exposes and confronts three deeply concerning and oppressive issues in our public school system:

First- A state of nearly absolute apartheid now prevails in thousands of our schools. The segregation of Black children has reverted to a level the nation has not seen since 1968. Fewer of the students in these schools know white children any longer.

Second- A protomilitary form of discipline has now emerged, modeled on stick-and-carrot methods of behavioral control traditionally used in prisons but targeted exclusively at Black and Hispanic children.

Third- As high-stakes testing takes on pathological and punitive dimensions, liberal education in our inner-city schools has been increasingly replaced by culturally barren and robotic methods of instruction that would be rejected out of hand by schools that serve the mainstream of society.

Ultimately, Kozol offers our nation a humane, dramatic challenge to fulfill, at last, the promise made some 50 years ago to all our youngest citizens.

Brown v. Board of Education

Brown v. Board of In 1954, the U.S. Supreme Court issued perhaps the most crucial decision in its history. At the heart of this decision was a powerful idea: students of different races will thrive together when they learn together.

Brown v. Board of Education of Topeka was a landmark decision of the U.S. Supreme Court in which the court ruled that U.S. state laws establishing racial segregation in public schools are unconstitutional, even if the segregated schools are otherwise equal in quality.

This milestone decision signaled the end of legalized racial segregation in the schools of the United States, overruling the "separate but equal" principle set forth in the 1896 Plessy v. Ferguson case. Determining that "separate but equal" schools for Afrikan-Americans and white students were unconstitutional ultimately opened the door to desegregating American schools.

Responses to the Brown v. Board of Education ruling ranged from enthusiastic approval to bitter opposition. The General Assembly adopted a policy of "Massive Resistance," using the law and the courts to obstruct desegregation.

Let us never forget that the Brown decision was propelled not merely by a principled objection to the idea of "separate but equal" but by Southern states' unrestrained contempt for the "equal" part of the formula. Black students were not only segregated but wholly denied meaningful educational opportunities.

The Topeka Brown case was crucial because it helped convince the court that even when physical facilities and other "tangible" factors were equal, segregation still deprived minority children of equal educational opportunities.

The legal victory in Brown did not transform the country overnight, and much work remains. However, striking down segregation in the nation's public schools provided a significant catalyst for the civil rights movement, making possible advances in desegregating housing, public accommodations, and institutions of higher education.

Conscious Assessment

The mere mention of apartheid schooling in America was concerning because I understood apartheid to be legalized discrimination. It is an ideology invented to establish strict control over economic and social systems and to maintain white domination while extending racial separation.

While traveling in South Afrika, I saw the effects of apartheid up close and in person. It has negatively affected the lives of all South Afrikan children, but its impact has been particularly devastating for Black children.

The consequences of poverty, racism, and violence have resulted in psychological disorders, producing a generation of maladjusted children resulting from this grossly inadequate and tragically implemented political divide.

Exposing these fundamental truths regarding this dreadful scheme is necessary because a state of nearly absolute apartheid schooling in America is unacceptable. However, the ideology of apartheid and the systemic challenges Afrikan Americans face within our public education system is not unique. They tell the same oppressive story with a different storyline.

Almost fifteen years later, recent studies still show gross underfunding of majority Black and Latino school districts, racially segregated schools, disproportionate disciplining of Black students, and curricula that reinforce racist ideology.

The state of education in Black America is complex and multidimensional. However, the most critical problem that Black America face is the gap in academic achievement between Blacks and Whites.

As our nation and schools become more diverse, the issue of closing the achievement gap becomes even more urgent. Let us also be mindful that the proportion of students of color in public schools has increased, and the enrollment rate constitutes a large percentage of the student population.

This assessment is significant because these proportional increases suggest that the prosperity of our nation will be increasingly dependent on the knowledge and contributions of students/children of color.

If the inequality in opportunity to learn and the disparity in achievement is ultimately to be eliminated, the nation must undertake a multifaceted initiative to improve the state of education for Black Americans.

We as a nation must develop a universal, well-rounded, and comprehensive curriculum for all students to establish and ensure a public education system in which all children participate, achieve at high levels, and reach their full potential.

We must also stabilize our communities' social fabric to protect better and support our children's academic and personal development, reducing the relatively high levels of academic under-achievement observed in many of our children and the schools that serve them.

Failing schools should be a reclamation project for the entire Black community. We must also be mindful that representation in all facets of life is crucial to the development of our communities.

Equally important, in our multifaceted roles as educators, policy-makers, parents, and community members, we must stimulate high levels of academic achievement for all students, particularly those our schools have least served.

Education is Key

Steven Pinker, a renowned Harvard University psychologist, describes the best educational focus for raising children who can succeed in their careers and be informed and responsible citizens:

> " A liberal education should make certain habits of rationality second nature. Educated people should be able to express complex ideas in clear writing and speech. They should appreciate that objective knowledge is a precious commodity and know how to distinguish vetted fact from superstition, rumor, and unexamined conventional wisdom. They should know how to reason logically and statistically, avoiding the fallacies and biases to which the untutored human mind is vulnerable. They should think causally rather than magically and know what it takes to

distinguish causation from correlation and coincidence. They should be acutely aware of human fallibility, most notably their own, and appreciate the value of trying to change minds by persuasion rather than intimidation or demagoguery... The more deeply a society cultivates this knowledge and mindset, the more it will flourish."

Education is arguably the ultimate equalizer. No matter what your socioeconomic status is, if you've got an education, you have power. Ultimately, the level and quality of educational attainment either opens the doors to opportunity or closes them.

Education is also the key to progress and prosperity in America today. Whether legitimate or not, educational opportunity and academic achievement are directly tied to the social divisions associated with race, ethnicity, gender, first language, and social class.

Therefore, we must understand that education starts at home, in neighborhoods, and in our communities. Further, as members of the Black community, we must take responsibility for educating all our children, whether ours by birth or otherwise, to uplift our people as a whole.

We as parents and elders must take the time to instill in our children a respect for education and an understanding of the power associated with attaining knowledge. This vital process of establishing, teaching, and nurturing is the beginning of their education for transformation.

Education for Transformation

When speaking of education for transformation, I'm speaking of the powerful information that is often not in most schools' curricula. Moreover, we must know, understand, and teach our children what culture is and why its crucial.

If you don't know your culture, anyone can tell you what your culture is and have you believing that the ways of your people are inferior. Culture is a weapon in a people's struggle because the suppression or denial of their culture is part of their enslavement.

Culture is also like the electricity that illuminates the light bulb. It is the vast structure of behaviors, ideas, attitudes, values, habits, beliefs, and practices peculiar to a particular group of people. It is also the invisible medium where all human functioning occurs; nothing happens outside of culture.

Ultimately, culture provides a general design for living and patterns for interpreting reality. It also has the power to compel behavior and give meaning to existence. In addition to understanding what culture is, it is essential to understand what racism is and how it affects all areas of people's activity.

Racism is prejudice plus power and functions as a result of fear and ignorance. As a powerful dynamic, it affects all areas of people's activity, including but not limited to economics, education, entertainment, labor, law, politics, religion, sex, and war.

We do not use racism as an excuse; however, it is highly pervasive. Racism is why we see so many economic and educational disparities, police brutality, and so much more. Though it is pervasive, we need not be dismayed or discouraged by racism.

Knowing our culture and honoring our Ancestral Obligations requires "a consciousness of victory" instead of dwelling on oppression. It requires that we tap into our personal and collective power, harness it and direct it toward transformative means.

Our personal and collective power is greater than racism once we awaken and unify, which is why so much energy is exerted in this society to keep us asleep, disunified, and disempowered.

Determination and Preparation

From the time of slavery to the present, Black Americans have struggled to attain high-quality education. During slavery, educating Blacks was forbidden. Today there is a legal right to attend school, but for many Blacks, a quality education is still challenging.

However, there is no hiding place from the realities, hardships, and challenges that reflect the complexity of Black survival and the mending of some long-lasting consequences.

Today's young Blacks are undoubtedly the most educated generation of Afrikan Americans in history. However, we must stop pretending our children are being prepared for the modern world because they aren't.

Education has become a big business for both the public and private industries. Public charter and some private schools compete eagerly for children; for some institutions, children are merely profit opportunities.

If we are ever going to have an educational breakthrough and fix our school system, our children must learn critical thinking methods early on and practice them throughout their educational process. They must be taught to question every premise, no matter who offers it.

Critical thinking methods teaches our children not just the individual subject matter but also how to continue to learn once they are out of school. Ultimately, this process is a vital step in developing certain habits of rationality as second nature even outside of liberal education.

The root of all evil in this world is arguably not the love of money but the addiction to illogical thinking because the perpetuation of ignorance comes with that. Our children must be taught to reason logically and statistically to avoid the fallacies and biases that young minds are vulnerable to.

Reading to our children, creating time and space for homework, engaging in enriching family and neighborhood activities for children of all ages, and demonstrating through words and actions that education is essential are fundamental building blocks for higher education.

If a dozen or more adults in any given community could adopt a school and spend one hour a week in the classroom, assisting the teacher or tutoring students, it would make a profound difference.

Elementary school students who lack proper motivation are more inclined to drop out of high school, which will affect their earning potential as adults hindering their ability to make a consistent financial contribution to their families.

Moreover, if a child lacks an appreciation for the educational process, the teacher will spend more time disciplining than teaching that child. School teachers can only reinforce that which a child brings to the classroom as a result of home training.

Equally important, while schools are responsible for what children are taught, parents are responsible for the reinforcement at home. One of the major problems in most school systems is the lack of parental involvement. Many parents have abdicated their responsibility to their children and the educational process.

We must understand that a solid and active parental organization will help determine what goes on in the classroom. We must also demand that local communities, state and federal governments provide the necessary resources to educate all children.

Think about this, if the effectiveness of education rests on such resources and they are unequally distributed, it is reasonable to anticipate that the effects of education will be unequal. More to the point, resources should be better invested in supporting our children's academic and personal maturity.

These resources must include supplemental enrichment programs because children's learning processes are enhanced by having forums to exercise other parts of their ongoing development.

The continuing development of parents is essential to ensure that they can advocate for and orchestrate the additional support necessary for the holistic development of their children. It is also the key to quality education.

The Hunt for Teachers

Many qualified, experienced teachers are no longer teaching, and addressing the teacher shortage shouldn't involve lowering the criteria to be a teacher. It should include supporting teachers, paying them, and providing the best resources to serve students.

In my opinion, there is no real teacher shortage. However, the pandemic made an already dire reality even more devastating. Research shows us that the gap in the number of available educators is most acute in areas including special education and educators who teach English language learners and substitutes.

More to the point, the real shortage is a lack of, or a need for, more respect for the craft, proper compensation, and teacher training, which the absence hinders the ability to teach effectively.

The bottom line remains; America will never correct its mistakes if teachers are not allowed to teach about them.

Ironically many say that history will judge—however, that isn't exactly a super compelling argument when some states are making it illegal to teach history.

Public Education in America is a vast subject with many tenets. However, Edmund W. Gordon sums it up quite well in his outstanding introductory essay _Establishing a System of Public Education._ He states with extreme certainty

"If we are actively engaged in our children's learning and development from an early age, and if we hold our elected officials responsible for providing well-rounded educational facilities, programs, and staff, then we can establish a system of public education in which all children participate, achieve at high levels, and reach their full potential. Education must be guaranteed as a civil right and civil liberty for every child in America."

We must never forget or always remember that an education is an investment in the future of not only the child but the entire family. So, either we contribute to the education of our children today, or our grandchildren will suffer tomorrow.

Ase (It is so)

Chapter 4
Identifying the Elements

In this chapter, I will objectively address and debate Critical Race Theory and how it intersects with varying forms of racism. Further, it will assist you in understanding the systemic challenges that have and will continue to negatively affect Afrikan American children for generations to come if not revealed and appropriately addressed.

As a nation, we proclaim that our fundamental political philosophy is to make our country fair and to fight every inequity so that all children can face their future with the same amount of hope, limited only by their vision and determination. More to the point, racism prevents that from being true.

In today's America, one of the most egregious and unfortunate results of growing up in a world wallpapered with racism is its effect on Black Children's self-images. With that being said, I'm reminded of the infamous "doll test." It has been conducted since the 1940s, revealing an early level of self-loathing in Black children.

In this doll test, young Black children are presented with a white doll and a Black doll and asked to choose which doll they like or would rather play with. A majority of the children choose the white doll. The white doll was often chosen when asked which was the nicest doll.

When one Black girl was asked why she chose the Black doll as the "bad" one, she said, "Because she's Black." The response is indicative of decades of racial and economic subordination. Without question, racism subverts the American ideal of a level playing field on which every child has an equal opportunity to succeed.

We must be mindful that to fix any problem or even come to a possible resolution, we must first and foremost understand the problem. Therefore, starting by establishing a fundamental understanding of racism is essential.

We must also understand that talking about racism is not an attempt to guilt or shame anyone. It is about spreading awareness so that it can be adequately addressed. Evoking change is a long process, but learning more about systemic racism is an essential first step.

The feminist political activist Angela Davis once said: *"In a racist society, it is not enough to be non-racist. We must be anti-racist."*

Unfortunately, the harsh reality is that there will never be an end to racism. However, Ibram Kendi states with extreme certainty that: *" To be antiracist is a radical choice in the face of history, requiring radical reorientation of our consciousness"*

Racism

Racism is prejudice plus the power to enforce one's bias. It is also a form of oppression in which one group dominates others, having the ability to impose systematic discrimination through the institutional policies and practices of society. Thereby shaping the cultural beliefs and values that support those racist policies and procedures.

In America, the dominant group is white; therefore, racism is white racial and cultural prejudice and discrimination by institutional power and authority used to the advantage of whites and the disadvantage of people of color.

Various types of racism negatively affect people of color, exploiting the racial divide. They include but are not limited to land ownership and housing, healthcare and medicine, criminal justice, and law enforcement, with overt and covert methods of implementation.

Structural/Institutional Racism

(Also called Systemic Racism) is distinguished from the explicit attitude or racial bias of individuals by the existence of systemic policies or laws and practices that provide differential access to goods, services, and opportunities of society by race.

Most of the rest of the world sees our unpleasant dilemma of racial disparity and uses it as a propaganda tool to damage our international reputation. Our enemies use it as a recruiting tool to enlist soldiers and terrorists.

Systemic Racism

Refers to the complex interactions of large-scale societal systems, practices, ideologies, and programs that produce and perpetuate inequities for racial minorities. So that even if individual racism is not present, adverse conditions and inequalities for racial minorities will continue to exist. In part, it even controls the mortality rate of minorities.

The life expectancy of Black men and women is lower than the life expectancy of white Americans. Because of the lack of high-quality options, Black babies die at a staggering rate, almost 2.5 times more often than white babies. Black women die three times more often than white women in childbirth. These are a few results of the systemic challenges Black people face.

Systemic means something is a big part of social, economic, or political practice. Unfortunately, we live in a world where a person's race and zip code are the most significant factors in determining their life expectancy. That is morally unacceptable.

Interpersonal Racism

(Also called Individual Racism or Personally Mediated Racism) is what most people think of when using the term racism. Individuals' beliefs, attitudes, and actions support or perpetuate racism. It can occur on multiple levels, conscious and unconscious, active and passive, and intentional and unintentional.

However, we must also acknowledge that racism is a practice and is not restricted to bad people. Let us also be mindful that change doesn't come from complaining or being morally right. It comes from the focused, persistent, intense confrontation of the problem.

Acknowledgment and Perpetuation of Oppression

While researching the Holocaust in late December 2019, I found that Germany is often praised for facing its Nazi past. However, the memory of the Holocaust is still up for debate. January 27, 2020, all eyes were on Germany as the world marked the 75th anniversary of the liberation of Auschwitz, a key part of a series of watershed World War II anniversaries.

More specifically, Germany's first female Chancellor, Angela Merkel, set the tone with a moving and highly reflective speech at the Auschwitz memorial in early December when she expressed a *"deep sense of shame for the barbaric crimes that Germans committed."*

The chancellor has come to embody how Germany has faced its Nazi past. As far as Germany's institutions and intellectuals are concerned, there exists a broad consensus that the country has confronted its crimes and learned its lessons.

Major cities boast impressive monuments, museums, and centers dedicated to the study of antisemitism and the Holocaust. Germany's institutions illustrate a conscious and responsible approach to dealing with its past sins.

To acknowledge means: to accept or admit the existence or truth of. On the other hand, perpetuation means the continuation or preservation of a situation, idea, etc. Some observers, including American philosophers, make the case that it's time for the rest of the world to begin "learning from the Germans."

Any system that deprives a people of its family structure denies the humanity of that people. History has no equal to match the horrific way in which white America (The Caucasian segment of America that advocates racial hatred and promotes social injustices) treated and destroyed the Black family.

More to the point, not only has America failed to acknowledge its transgressions against Black people, America has continued perpetuating oppression through systemic racism. We must acknowledge and denounce the systemic perpetuation of racism and social injustices enacted upon Black people throughout our nation's history.

Only then will we as a nation be able to rise up and live out the true meaning of our creed; we hold these truths to be self-evident that all men are created equal.

Critical Race Theory (CRT)

Is Critical Race Theory (CRT) a way of understanding how American racism has shaped public policy or a divisive discourse that pits people of color against white people?

Fundamentally, the disagreement stems from different conceptions of racism. However, CRT emphasizes outcomes, not merely on an individual's beliefs, and it calls on these outcomes to be examined and rectified.

After extensive research and an astute understanding of Critical Race Theory, I have concluded that CRT is not a divisive discourse that pits people of color against white people; it is much more than just pointing to race. Further, understanding Critical Race Theory requires engaging and articulating the material, structural, and ideological mechanisms of white supremacy.

Critical Race Theory (CRT) is an academic concept over fifty years old. The core idea is that race is a social construct, and racism is not just the product of individual bias or prejudice but is embedded in legal systems and policies. CRT primarily examines social, cultural, and legal issues related to race and racism in our nation.

Another crucial tenet of CRT is that racism and specific racial outcomes result from complex, changing, and often subtle social and institutional dynamics in conjunction with the explicit and intentional prejudices that affect people of color.

The basic tenets of Critical Race Theory emerged out of a framework for legal analysis in the late 1970s and early 1980s. They were created by legal scholars Derrick Bell, Kimberle Crenshaw, and Richard Delgado, who sought to examine the intersection of race and law in America and challenge the mainstream approaches to racial justice.

UCLA Law School's <u>CRT Forward Tracking Project</u> has tracked 567 anti-critical race theory (CRT) efforts introduced at the local, state, and federal levels. According to the *World Population Review*, there are currently seven states that have banned CRT, while another 16 states are in the process of banning it. That constitutes almost all states with a Republican governor.

Most of the current laws are targeting public institutions in Republican-controlled states because they are part of a national agenda. House Speaker, Kevin McCarthy pledged to fix "woke education indoctrination in our schools," while former President Donald Trump has made the "issue" a priority for his 2024 campaign.

They want to stimulate "patriotic education" but cut federal funding for any school or program that includes "critical race theory, gender ideology, or other inappropriate racial, sexual, or political content unto our children." And university administrators will not risk losing millions of federal funding for a "gender" or "race" class, not even at the private Ivy Leagues in solidly blue states.

While CRT is a highly specific academic theory that is almost exclusively taught at some law schools, the anti-CRT laws are incredibly broad and vague, targeting all levels of education. Here in Georgia, *House Bill 1084* bans the use of so-called divisive concepts from teaching. However, it includes several exceptions and stipulations that are so broad and vague that many teachers will simply stay away from these divisive concepts.

All bills explicitly ban the teaching of classic racism, "one race is superior to another race." They have also banned the teaching of institutional or structural racism, "the idea racial discrimination is not just the consequence of a few racist individuals, it is structural, engrained in the country's key institutions – from election laws to law enforcement."

The idea is simple and obvious: if children are not taught about institutional racism, and the white supremacy it upholds, they won't question it later when they are voters. This practice is a classic case of historical revisionism. How we see the past determines our future.

To counter the highly organized conservative attack, we need a concerted and integrated campaign/effort from all individuals and organizations that support academic freedom and liberal democracy.

The Five Basic Tenets of CRT - The Core Components

The importance of experiential knowledge. CRT says that the lived experiences of people of color, however, expressed (storytelling, family history, biographies, parables, narratives), are crucial to understanding racism and oppression, and they are necessary in our quest for liberation. From the academic to legal to the activist arenas, the lived experience must be taken seriously.

We must understand that only those who have been successfully mis-educated have no desire to know their past. However, it is essential because history illuminates the safest path before us by revealing the pitfalls of the past.

Without question, history is open to interpretation. However, it is crucial for all children, particularly Black children, to understand that history can be a critical guide to their present and future, both personally and culturally.

The centrality and intersectionality of racism. Racism exists everywhere in American life –from within our own thoughts, to our personal relationships, to our places of work, to our educational and judicial systems. CRT says that racism isn't just the actions of individuals but is embedded in our institutions, systems, and culture. It is our way of life.

The challenge to dominant ideology. In law and other arenas there is a belief that concepts like neutrality, objectivity, colorblindness, and meritocracy can be fully actualized. CRT says, how can one be truly neutral on issues of race when racism is baked into the fabric of America?

In a 2007 U.S. Supreme Court school-assignment case on whether race could be a factor in maintaining diversity in K-12 schools, Chief Justice John Roberts' opinion concluded:

"The way to stop discrimination on the basis of race is to stop discriminating on the of basis race." But during oral arguments, then-Justice Ruth Bader Ginsburg said: *"It's very hard for me to see how you can have a racial objective but a nonracial means to get there."*

CRT pointed out that claims of objectivity and colorblindness can be ways in which dominant groups camouflage their interests to get what's best for them. Housing and education are prime examples in this country.

The commitment to social justice. CRT, as a framework, acknowledges how all oppression interrelates and focuses on eradicating racism and other forms of oppression by centering people of color and taking a stance on issues of social justice.

Moreover, people of color have been fighting before this country was formed for justice in some form or fashion, which has never stopped.

The use of an interdisciplinary perspective. CRT draws from many different fields to create a powerful and nuanced framework for engaging with race and racism. There is no one answer, no one discipline, and no one path to freedom. CRT says let's use all the tools in the toolbox to help educate folks so we can get free.

CRT is more theoretical than I have described, but this is it at its core. It is rooted in collective learning and community building. It is also an education that values challenging the status quo and prioritizing lived experiences. CRT is the education that most of us only got after leaving school.

Critical Race Theory- Ties

CRT also has ties to other intellectual currents, including the works of sociologists and literary theorists who studied links between political power, social organizations, and languages. Equally notable, its ideas have since informed other fields, such as the humanities, the social sciences, and teacher education.

CRT reveals a way of understanding how our nation's racism has shaped public policy. An appropriate example is when, in the 1930s, government officials drew lines around areas deemed a poor financial risk, often explicitly due to the racial composition of the inhabitants. As a result, banks refused to offer mortgages to Black people in those areas.

This behavior is a prime example of institutional racism, also known as systemic racism. Today, those same patterns of discrimination live on through race-blind policies, like single-family zoning that prevents the building of affordable housing in advantaged, majority-white neighborhoods and, thus, hindering racial desegregation efforts.

These patterns refer to the ongoing racial inequities maintained and embedded in the laws and regulations of society, manifesting as discrimination in criminal justice, employment, health care, education, and political representation.

Further, data regarding systemic racism vividly show the racial divide across every system. For families of color and their children, it determines where they live, the quality of the education they receive, their income, the type of food they have access to, and their overall exposure to societal opportunities.

Critical Race Theory in Education

This topic has exploded in the public arena regarding education, especially K-12, where numerous state legislatures are debating bill seeking to ban its use in classrooms. Others believe it is a divisive discourse that pits people of color against white people.

Critical Race Theory studies in education could be defined as a critique of racism as a system of oppression and exploitation that explores the historical and contemporary constructions and manifestations of race in our society with particular attention to how these issues are manifested in schools.

Scholars who study Critical Race Theory regarding education look at how policies and practices in K-12 education contribute to continued racial inequalities in education and advocate ways to change them.

Their studies included but weren't limited to racially segregated schools, the underfunding of majority-Black and Latino school districts, disproportionate disciplining of Black students, barriers to gifted programs, selective-admission high schools, and curricula that reinforce racist ideology.

Within the last two decades, CRT has become an increasingly permanent fixture in the toolkit of education researchers seeking to critically examine educational opportunities, school climate, representation, and the method and practice of teaching.

Ultimately, scholars have looked to CRT as a tool to help analyze the experiences of historically underrepresented populations across the K-20 educational pipeline.

K-12 Teaching and Learning

Another critical issue explored by researchers utilizing CRT in education is teaching. This area examines teacher attitudes, behaviors, and practices. CRT theorists analyzing teaching often deal with subjectivity and how teacher subjectivities motivate them to engage in issues important to Critical Race curricular and pedagogical approaches.

Research that utilizes CRT to examine teaching finds that a critical aspect of teacher attitudes mimics larger problematic ideologies such as colorblindness, meritocracy, and liberal attitudes that see race as an individualized issue.

The composition of teachers is an important question addressed by Critical Race scholars. Research shows a need for teachers of color. Research also tells us that teachers are most effective when they teach in ways that are culturally relevant to students of color.

Being culturally relevant is more than knowing a student's culture; it extends to understanding that students' cultures operate in a historical and contemporary context where white supremacy institutionalizes a hierarchy in which whites are at the top. People of color are at the bottom.

CRT helps to expose this reality by examining teacher attitudes and practices while simultaneously offering mechanisms to move such limiting attitudes and practices toward more liberating ends.

For a more conclusive and in-depth understanding of Critical Race Theory in education, I highly recommend reading: *Critical Race Theory in Education: A Review of Past Literature and a Look to the Future.* Maria C. Ledesma, Dolores Calderon, First Publisher February 25, 2015.

This article examines the development of Critical Race Theory in education, paying attention to how researchers use CRT (and its branches) in studying K-12 and higher education. The article reviews CRT literature focusing on CRT scholarship that offers tools to engage with and work against racism within education.

The authors highlight works that embody the critical origins of CRT in both the law and elsewhere to demonstrate that CRT work means more than just pointing to race. It requires an engagement and articulation with the material, structural, and ideological mechanisms of white supremacy.

Those who don't or won't understand the radical reorientation of Critical Race Theory will continue contributing to the perpetuation of inequality, broken promises, and betrayal of our children.

Practical Proposal

Providing equal education for children in all income brackets is a practical proposal that offers some relief. Unquestionably, a good education is one of the best roads to escaping the cycle of poverty, but for many Children of color, that's a false hope.

The dropout rate among low-income families is seven times more than families with higher incomes. Forty percent of impoverished children are not adequately prepared to attend primary school. As a result, by the end of 4th grade, Afrikan-American, Latino, and low-come students are two years behind grade level; by 12th grade, they are four years behind, and money is a massive part of the problem.

Impoverished children don't get an equal share of the educational funds. Recent and prior reports from the U.S. Department of Education conclude that more than 40 percent of low-income schools don't get as much state and local funds as schools serving higher-income families.

Because there are so many more challenges for schools with low-income students, it makes more sense for such schools to receive more money, not less, but that is not the reality. "WHY?"

Shem Hotep (I go in peace)

Chapter 5
Body Talk

The human body is truly a wondrous creation and a miracle to behold. It is unequaled in its complexity and unlimited in its potential. Moreover, the body is even more ingenious when we realize that all body cells are replaced every twelve months. What a phenomenal opportunity we're given to recreate what we inherited!

However, the body is still a projection of the mind, and only by educating the mind can we seize this opportunity mother nature has given us. More specifically, this process does not happen by chance or overnight.

You need a vision, a plan, and a personal commitment to follow a lifestyle of regular exercise, nutritious eating, proper rest, and a positive state of mind. Herein lies the foundation of health, fitness, and wellness.

This concept is essential for us to understand as a people and even more crucial for children of color, particularly

Afrikan/American children, due to our past. Let us also be mindful that the door of wisdom is never closed. Therefore, we must learn from yesterday, live today, and plan for tomorrow.

My Story

I now understand that humanity is designed to be spiritually aware, emotionally alert, mentally creative, physically fit, and continually striving to achieve goals. I am ultimately acknowledging that fitness is a state of mind.

With over 40 years of experience in the fitness industry, I offer optimal training programs ranging from flexibility training, weight training, dietary manipulation, therapeutic modalities, biomechanical skill training, and nutritional supplementation.

More to the point, I am a living inspiration and testament to how a healthy lifestyle can help win battles over ailments and dreadful diseases. In September 1993, at age 35, the peak of my life, I stood toe to toe with adversity. I suffered a heart attack secondary to blocked arteries and underwent a five-artery bypass surgery.

This life-changing experience devastated my family and me. Never could I imagine anything like this happening to me. But with faith and iron will, I exclaimed, "I will not be defeated!" My primary motivation was based on the fact that my family needed me.

Unless someone has experienced this type of trauma they cannot imagine the physical, emotional, spiritual, and financial toll these dreaded diseases take on a family's life. I credit my success in this challenging surgery and recovery to the grace of God and my mental, physical, and spiritual conditioning.

Without those attributes, my chances of surviving the heart attack and surgery would have been slim to none. Exercising for overall fitness has become a way of life for me because I've learned that the benefits outweigh the consequences of not exercising or adopting that way of life.

My family history of heart disease and cancer made it incumbent upon me to do extensive research regarding physical fitness associated with decreased risk of illness and death. Numerous studies showed low fitness is associated with a shorter life span. Other studies found that physical fitness reduced the risk of death from cancer and heart disease, among other illnesses.

After extensive research, the choice became clear. My heart had been opened on an anatomical level; now, I have learned how to open it on multiple levels. I also had to learn how to feel freer and happier, a different kind of open heart procedure; one based on love, knowledge, and compassion rather than just drugs and surgery.

I've made the connection between when I feel stressed and why; then, stress became my teacher instead of my enemy. I stopped viewing pain (physical, emotional, and spiritual) as punishment and began seeing it as information.

Spiritual Symbolism of the Body

After understanding the spiritual symbolism of the different parts of the body, I realized that besides the physical function is the spiritual function, which is carrying on a parallel activity in the invisible.

Physical activity is merely the visible, factual expression of the inner reality. The real care of the body is done on the spiritual level. No part of the body is isolated from the whole.

Our body is the physical expression of an integrated and united organism, which includes the mental, emotional, and spiritual levels. Let us take a look at the spiritual correspondence of the human body.

Head Body

Head	Awareness	Back	Support
Mind	Reason	Body	Manifestation
Nerves	Communication	Chest	Potential
Brain	Thought	Hand	Attention/Grasp
Face	Recognition	Fingers	Persistence
Eyes	Perception	Fingernails	Examination
Ears	Understanding/Balance/Faith	Thumb	Comparison
Nose	Direction	Wrist	Freedom
Teeth	Analysis	Arm	Action
Mouth	Praise and Thanksgiving	Elbow	Movement

Tongue	Appreciation	Shoulder	Power
Skin	Protection/ Individuality	Leg	Forward movement
Voice	Communication	Knee	Variety
Throat	Expression	Ankle	Ease
Breath	Life	Heel	Conviction
Neck	Flexibility	Toes	Concentration
Hair	Vitality/Strength	Toenails	Details

The human body is, without question, the most exquisite and wonderful organization which has come from the divine hands.

Learning From Yesterday/Our Story

To truly learn from yesterday, we must revisit the triumphs and tragedies of our story. First and foremost, thank God for bringing us through some of the most horrific experiences enslaved Black people suffered. My sisters and brothers know that our God was with our Ancestors as he is with us. He has a work planned for us.

After the Afrikan was seized and taken from his homeland and family, he experienced a tragic trip across the Atlantic Ocean. This trip set a trend of horrific experiences that would affect his health and the health of his descendants for generations to come.

Once in America and on the plantation, the Black slaves developed bad health habits and lifestyles because rigid schedules with limited resources were forced on them. The

Black slave had little time to sleep, inadequate meals, unbelievably stressful situations, and many other experiences that contributed to bad health.

More to the point, our survival experience has left some lasting consequences on Blacks' health and health habits in America. The health habits and lifestyles forced upon enslaved Blacks became tradition. The consequences of these traditions are still affecting the health status of Blacks today.

Sadly, today some of these killers are called cultural. Once a habit or behavior becomes cultural, the group usually defends the habit/behavior. However, we must no longer defend bad health and make sure our children know the difference.

Living for Today/Lifestyle Change

When I initially heard the word "generational curse" associated with bad health regarding Black people, I was terrified simply because of the negative connotation surrounding the word curse, but the reality was even more frightening.

The generational curse refers to the perpetuation of the health habits and lifestyle forced on Black slaves that still affect the health of Black people today. Black Americans must look closely at their lifestyle and health habits, only keeping healthy behaviors and practices while eliminating those indicative of bad health.

Everyone has their barriers to change. However, several ways exist to overcome these barriers and make lifestyle changes. One crucial way to overcome these barriers is knowing that knowledge is a vital motivational tool for making behavioral changes.

We all have reasons that are especially important and powerful enough to get us going; even when we're not in the mindset, you need to find out what these reasons are for you.

Many environmental and personal factors can help overcome barriers to making change. Reinforcement is one of the essential factors which can lead to either a positive or negative consequence of behavior.

Positive reinforcement is a reward that you gain as a result of making progress toward a goal. In contrast, negative reinforcement is a negative consequence to help you get moving in the right direction.

In addition to understanding the importance of reinforcement, you should be aware that you may have limits. Ultimately, to facilitate change, you must not only believe that you can make the change happen, but you must also work at making the change.

Another point to consider when making lifestyle changes is that behavior can be influenced by personal beliefs and feelings as well as the surrounding environment. This scenario includes being around people who want to achieve similar goals as you.

Ways to improve your environment include getting an exercise buddy, joining an exercise group, or hiring a personal trainer. The best way to improve your health is to develop behaviors associated with a healthy lifestyle. Minor changes are the first steps toward overall behavior change and improving your life.

Planning for Tomorrow/Preparing Our Children

As stated earlier, we as parents and elders must take the time to instill in our children a respect for education and an understanding of the power associated with attaining knowledge. This vital process of establishing, teaching, and nurturing is the beginning of their education for transformation.

Planning for tomorrow is synonymous with preparing our children for the future. Gone are the days when one graduated from high school, got a job, and pursued the American Dream. Now there is a new direction children of color, particularly Black children, must take to achieve self-fulfillment and success.

A healthy lifestyle accompanied by higher education is now the required catalyst to launch the pursuit of most dreams. A healthy lifestyle and education should be prioritized in our children's lives.

A healthy lifestyle is imperative while in school because it is the basic guideline for a lifetime of healthy living. Further, establishing good health, fitness, and wellness are the keys to a healthy lifestyle.

More specifically, they all emphasize self-responsibility for a lifestyle process that realizes the individual's highest physical, mental, and spiritual well-being. This process will prepare our children to participate fully in life, to be free from controllable health risk factors, and to achieve mental and physical objectives consistent with their potential.

Health-Fitness-and-Wellness

Let's take time to understand the components of a healthy lifestyle:

Health is the overall condition of an organism at a given time. In addition to soundness of mind and body, free from disease or abnormality.

Fitness is the state or condition of being physically sound and healthy from exercise and proper nutrition.

Wellness is the condition of good physical and mental health when adequate diet, exercise, and habits are maintained. Wellness also encompasses a unique set of dimensions/skills that make a healthy lifestyle necessary for our children. They help create vision, balance, accountability, and commitment. These dimensions/skills of wellness are:

Emotional-The ability to control stress and express emotions appropriately and comfortably.

Intellectual-The ability to learn and use information effectively.

Occupational- The ability to balance work/school and leisure in a way that promotes health and a sense of personal satisfaction.

Physical- The physical component of wellness involves the ability to carry out daily tasks, developing cardio-respiratory, muscular fitness, and maintaining adequate nutrition.

Social-The ability to interact successfully with people and one's environment.

Spiritual-The spiritual component of wellness provides meaning and direction in life and enables us to grow, learn and meet new challenges.

Environmental- The environmental component of wellness includes promoting health measures that improve the community standard of living and quality of life, including laws and agencies that safeguard the physical environment.

Regular Exercise

To make exercise a way of life, we must go one step further. In our ancient Afrikan culture and tradition, exercise was a tool used to harness an even greater potential than the physical skills derived directly from it.

Exercise was designed to take the integrated mind, body, and spirit established at rest into dynamic physical activity and then into daily life. In layman's terms, exercise is a process and product of relaxation, rejuvenation, and mind and body coordination.

Clients often come to me wanting to start a fitness program for a special upcoming event or just to lose a few unwanted pounds acquired over time. Women's primary concern is that they don't want to get bulky from weightlifting; conversely, men want to bulk up. Other objectives are just to maintain.

Achieving Fitness Goals

The common denominator in achieving fitness goals, particularly changing your body, is understanding, adjusting, and readjusting body metabolism. Body metabolism is simply the rate at which the body burns its way through calories to keep itself alive, to keep the heart beating, the lungs breathing, the blood pumping, and the mind fantasizing.

Three types of calorie burns that happen throughout the day:

1. <u>The Thermic Effect of Eating</u>-Between 10-30 percent of the calories you burn each day gets burned by the act of digesting your food.

2. <u>Exercise and Movement</u>-Another 10-15 percent of your calorie burn comes from moving your muscles.

3. <u>Basal Metabolism or Resting Metabolism</u>-Refers to the calories you burn when you're doing nothing. Moreover, between 60-80 percent of your daily calories are burned just doing nothing because your body is constantly in motion.

Essential Components for Changing Body Metabolism

1. <u>Aerobic Exercise</u>-Essentially burns only at the time of the workout.

2. <u>Anaerobic/Strength Training</u>-Burns calories long after you leave the gym, while you sleep, and maybe until your next workout. Additionally, the extra muscle you build through strength training means your body keeps burning calories at rest to keep the new muscles alive.

3. <u>Dietary Manipulation and Supplementation</u>-Protein is the most versatile player on the nutrient team. It is critical for helping the body function at optimum levels.

Protein builds the framework of your body, including muscle, organs, bones, and connective tissues. It comes in many forms and does so many things well.

Carbohydrates are the body's primary source of raw material for energy. However, carbs are a double edge sword.

The best carbs are those foods that are grown and rich in fiber. The bad carbs trigger the release of excess insulin, make you fat and lethargic and cause hypoglycemia (low blood sugar), hunger, craving, and overeating, just to mention a few side effects.

Fat is among the most underrated and misunderstood of all the nutrient team members. Fat is not always the villain; it also acts as a secondary source of energy during training.

Fat base energy becomes available soon after carbohydrates stored in your muscles deplete. Even though carbs are your body's primary energy source, fats are the most highly concentrated source of energy over carbs and protein.

These essential fatty acids aid in many bodily functions, including the regulation of blood pressure and cholesterol in your blood. These essential fats are also classified as either monounsaturated fats or polyunsaturated fats.

Understanding the dietary importance of water is crucial. Water makes up 70-75 percent of your body weight, and your food also contains about 70 percent water. A 10 percent reduction of water in your body can make you sick, and a loss of 20 percent can mean death.

Water is involved in every bodily function known to man. Your vital fluid, blood, is comprised of 90 percent water. The importance of water is unquestionable as a significant "ingredient" of the human body. Adequate water is essential to health.

Stress Management- The component or group of skills for dealing with the stress imposed on an individual without suffering psychological distress and physical disorders.

Stress is the human response to overstimulation and has been linked with almost every medical problem known to man, including but not limited to heart attacks, strokes, hypertension, ulcers, colitis, asthma, arthritis, and cancer.

To understand stress and how to manage it, we must recognize a critical distinction between stressors and stress.

Stressors refer to the outside forces we must deal with. Stress refers to the individual's response to the stressors.

Ultimately, it is not what we must deal with (stressors) but rather how we deal with it (response) that dictates the severity of stress in our lives. Freedom from stress or the group of skills for coping with stress includes:

1. Meditation 2. Laughing 3. Proper planning and organization 4. Positive mental attitude 5. Commitment to cause 6. Adequate rest 7. Liberal use of water (inside & out)

Simple lifestyle changes, psychological assistance, medical support, and exercise all stand out as significant stress-controlling technologies.

It is essential that Black children are included in the conversation regarding "Body Talk." Understanding that habits tie us down, good or bad, and our lifestyles are often little more than the sum of our habits, and we determine our destiny by the choices we make each day.

How our children think or feel shapes their character and their choices make physical and chemical changes in their brains that send messages through the rest of the body through nerve cells; in this process, thoughts form actions, and repeated actions form habits.

Proverbs 22:6 says, "Train up a child in the way he should go: and when he is old, he will not depart from it."

Children spend approximately seven hours a day in school absorbing knowledge and being trained to apply it to their lives. Therefore, a school should be the place that greatly influences a child's life. Unfortunately, for many children of color, it's not.

In essence, the school should be a foundation for health and education. Healthy lifestyle education in schools could foster a profound reduction in risk factors associated with many diseases.

Encouraging and incorporating healthy eating, exercise, stress reduction, and coping skills in our schools is a crucial first step. Teaching children the importance of caring for themselves in a multi-faceted way makes for healthier adults in the future.

Separating Myth From Fact

m- Aerobics is better for shaping up than weight training.
F- To transform your physique, you must train with weights.

m- If you exercise, it doesn't matter what you eat.
F- If you exercise, it matters even more what you eat.

m- If women lift weights, they'll get "Bulky."
F- Resistance exercises help women create lean, toned bodies.

m- Weight training is only for young athletes.
F- People of all ages should be weight trained.

m- Muscles grow while you're working out.
F- Muscles grow while you're resting and recuperating.

m- A certain number of sets and reps gets the job done.
F- High-intensity effort produces the best results.

m- Eating right means three "square meals" a day.
F- Eating six nutritious meals a day is the right way.

m- People who overeat lack willpower.
F- Overeating is a natural instinct.

m- High-carbohydrate, low-fat diets work best.
F- People are becoming fat from a "carb. overdose."

m- You have to count every calorie you eat.
F- You should count "portions," not calories.

m- If you "eat right," you don't need to take supplements.
F- Studies show many of us do need to take supplements.

m- You need to drink water only when you are thirsty.
F- Your body needs more water than it's telling you.

m- You have to eat "perfectly" all the time.
F- There's no such thing as eating "perfectly."

Five Steps to Creating a Positive Cycle in Your Life

<u>Exercise aerobically and anaerobically</u>- Four to five times a week (preferably in the morning). Exercise in the zone(70-80 percent of your target heart rate).

<u>Eat a low-fat, balanced diet daily</u>- Eat six nutritious meals daily. Have at least two servings of fruit and three servings of vegetables daily.

<u>Drink six to eight glasses of water daily</u>- Limit or eliminate alcohol.

<u>Stop eating two to three hours before bedtime.</u>

<u>Review your commitment to healthy living daily.</u>

Renewing yourself is more than a step. It is a philosophy- an outlook on life. It's an intergraded approach to creating a positive cycle in your life. It's a way to remind yourself of your goals and what you are willing or going to do to work toward achieving them.

Daily renewal begins when you first wake up. Take a few moments to state what is important to you, what you wish to accomplish, and the steps you will take to work toward your goals that day.

Each evening, take the time to review how your day went. You will have one of two positive results. 1. You meet your challenge. 2. If your challenge is not met, you give yourself the opportunity to improve.

The body is indeed an instrument, the most sacred instrument, an instrument that God himself has made for His divine purpose. If it is kept in tune and the strings are not allowed to become loose, this instrument becomes the means of that harmony for which God created man.

Nehas (The Awakening)

Chapter 6
Preparing Our Children

In preparing our children for the future, we must grasp where we are now because this is where we, as a people (Afrikan Americans), can establish ourselves as an invaluable part of society. If not, we risk becoming a permanent underclass with decreasing influence.

Afrikan Americans face devastating disparities on nearly every imaginable level, from health to housing, crime to criminal justice, and education to economic parity. However, the time has come for us to shift the conversation from acknowledging the pain and devastation to developing a plan of radical reorientation for the sake of our children.

First and foremost, we must acknowledge that parental involvement is still one of the most significant contributions to the academic and overall social success of Afrikan American children/students. Therefore, it is necessary for us, as parents, to instill in our children a respect for education and an understanding of the power associated with the attainment of knowledge.

This power will not only allow our children to know and understand that they have a role in creating the world they want for generations to come, but it will also allow them to be active participants in the creation process. Only then will we be able to move toward the days we dream of when justice and morality are the norms instead of just an aspiration for the future?

The Changing World

Today, almost every job requires technical skills or computer knowledge, and the world's need for technology will continue to grow, creating endless opportunities. Over the last decade, there's been much discussion surrounding Black participation in digital technology.

Numerous studies and reports have exposed the gap between Blacks and whites in computer ownership and internet access. Incidentally, both are essential subjects and are fundamental in scope.

Global forces in technology, research, science, and telecommunications make it clear that the future won't hold much promise for generations of Blacks if the trends that limit Afrikan American participation in the global digital technology economy aren't reversed.

It is imperative for Afrikan Americans to close the gap between computer ownership, access to broadband internet, and computer and technology literacy to participate and compete in the digital economy.

Furthermore, we must ensure that the quality of education in our children's schools plays a meaningful role in allowing and preparing them to adequately compete in a world of technology and embrace the digital economy. Now is the time to advocate for change within our schools, businesses, and communities because unpredictable global changes are rapidly occurring.

The Gap

The Internet is arguably the single most powerful and influential information source and educational tool ever invented. The digital divide describes the gap between people who have access to affordable, reliable internet service and the skills and gadgets necessary to take advantage of that access and those who don't.

The digital divide encompasses the technical and financial ability to utilize available technology, along with access or the lack of access to the internet as well as access to other forms of digital communication.

However, the divide exists in countless ways, including but not limited to urban and rural areas, developed and under-developed countries, ethnic groups, men and women even ocean-bordering and landlocked countries.

The access divide is the most visible digital divide regarding Black people, particularly our children. It refers to the socioeconomic differences among people and the impact on their ability to afford the devices necessary to get online.

The use divide refers to the difference in the level of skill individuals possess, which is affected by the quality of education an individual receives. The quality-of-use gap refers to the different ways people use the internet and the fact that some people are far more able to get the information they need from it than others.

These gaps reflect differences in wealth and access to education, as well as gender and racial discrimination. The digital divide also exacerbates these differences by barring many people from the information necessary to change their lives.

The global digital divide was seen as a consequence of economic development. More to the point, incomes have risen worldwide over the past decades, and access to digital services has remained low in much of the developing world.

In part, this is due to a need for more investment in internet infrastructure. Moreover, the internet penetration rate varies widely among continents: In 2022, 80% of Europeans had internet access, compared with just 22% of Afrikans.

Consequences of the Digital Divide

Technological discrimination is a form of social exclusion because it deprives certain people, particularly Black people, of essential resources for wealth development. This consensus is most visible when we look at the balance of the world economy, particularly the rapid growth in the number of jobs requiring digital access and skills.

In the U.S., nearly half of all careers in STEM (science, technology, engineering, and math) are in computing. Lack of access to learning these skills is a barrier to these jobs and the income that comes with them.

Consequences of the digital divide include isolation, which has affected mental health, increased educational barriers as education increasingly moves online, and worsening gender and racial exclusion/ discrimination.

The COVID-19 pandemic has brought into focus the isolation people without internet access or skills can experience and add barriers to education. As a result, children of color may have even more significant educational gaps.

The Coronavirus pandemic has also exposed the differences in digital coverage in the U.S. among children forced to attend school remotely and in less affluent communities.

The impact of this phenomenon has reached and is presently affecting people of color in devastating ways.

Narrowing the Digital Divide

Recently, programs have been launched to combat particular aspects of the digital divide. More to the point, it is incumbent upon societies to address the digital range holistically, recognizing its many elements and adverse outcomes.

November 15, 2021, President Joe Biden signed the bipartisan Infrastructure Investment and Jobs Act into law. It includes $65 billion for narrowing the digital divide. This multifaceted bill aims at reducing the digital divide by bringing high-speed internet to rural areas in America. It mandates that the Federal Communications Commission must adopt rules prohibiting digital redlining.

Within the bill is the Digital Equity Act, which establishes two new federal grant programs "to promote digital equality nationwide."

The state government will run one program and provide state-by-state digital equity planning followed by implementation grants to qualifying programs. The other program creates a yearly national competitive grant program "to support digital equity projects undertaken by individual groups, coalitions, and communities of interest anywhere in the U.S."

Ultimately, it is incumbent upon us as Black parents to ensure that every Black child understands that the world is becoming a technology-driven place. The number of Black students/youth prepared to participate in the higher levels of technology must be increased.

More specifically, young Blacks entering an information-based, technology-driven marketplace without the necessary technical skill sets will not only be unemployable, they will also be irrelevant.

Reclaiming Our Democracy

Today, at a time of bipartisan support for creating a multi-ethnic democracy in Ukraine and across the globe, it seems that we have forgotten about our need for bipartisan support for multi-ethnic democracy right here at home.

We, the people, particularly Afrikan/American people must understand that voting is one of the most important rights of American citizens because it empowers us to make choices. More specifically, voting is our ethical, moral, and political voice. It's also our voice for change, which must be heard.

Voting is also our opportunity to determine the distribution of political power. Our sacred responsibility and a joyful right that can enhance our lives for generations to come. Further, it is essential that our children are taught and understand how crucial voting rights are and the price our Ancestors paid to get them.

Let us boldly and humbly acknowledge our Ancestors' many sacrifices that have forced our nation to acknowledge and move toward adhering to its promises of democracy and equality regarding Afrikan Americans and voting rights.

However, while basking blissfully in our Ancestors' accomplishments, let us not forget how far we still must go to achieve full equality. We must also acknowledge the need to reauthorize further and strengthen the law to get there.

Ironically, America has one of the lowest voting rates among developed countries. More to the point, Afrikan

Americans were almost disenfranchised in this country for quite some time. A significant part of the lack of desire to vote particularly stems from the feeling of being deprived.

The poor, minorities and the young often feel overwhelmed and insignificant in the face of the political machine that seems indifferent to them. However, when these groups become a powerful voting bloc, politicians will aggressively count on them, and laws to help them will become more of a priority.

And to add insult to injury, these unfortunate indifferences are by intentional design and manifested through deception and persuasion. We should refrain from deceiving or persuading our people/children to vote. We must teach them the wisdom of voting based on self-interest. Ultimately, we must "Teach," not deceive or persuade.

The New Beginning

When most people think of patriotism, they often associate it with fighting on a foreign battlefield. Still, it can also be associated with fighting on the domestic battlefield. Voting rights for Afrikan Americans have been central on the domestic battlefield for some time.

It's a struggle that Afrikan Americans know all too well. A battle we were intentionally engaged in without our knowledge or consent. Ironically, this fight has made Afrikan Americans some of the most patriotic citizens of this country because they fight for what best serves the ideals of the Constitution. If that isn't patriotism, then what is?

The path to full voting rights for all American citizens has been long and often challenging. Originally under the Constitution, only white male citizens over 21 could vote. Fortunately, this shameful injustice has been corrected, and voting rights have been extended several times throughout our history.

Before the Civil War, and even after the enactment of the Fifteenth Amendment of the Constitution in 1870, which gave all men–regardless of race, color, or previous condition of ser-vitude–the right to vote, states still found ways to circumvent the Constitution and prevent Blacks from voting.

Almost a century later, the Voting Rights Act of 1965 was enacted. It is a landmark piece of federal legislation in the United States that prohibits racial discrimination in voting. Often cited as the most successful civil rights statute ever enacted.

The Voting Rights Act of 1965 (VRA) aimed to overcome legal barriers at the state and local level that prevented Afri-kan Americans from exercising their right to vote as guaranteed under the Fifteenth Amendment of the Constitution.

This time in history was truly a new beginning for Afrikan American/Black citizens. For the first time, the federal government required states to comply with the Fifteenth Amendment of the Constitution.

Today, citizens over 18 cannot be denied the right to vote on the basis race, religion, sex, disability, or sexual orientation, except for North Dakota. As a result, America is a better place today than in 1965 because of the Voting Rights Act. Since 1965, Afrikan American registration and turnout rates have increased dramatically.

Additionally, there are fifty-nine members of the Congressional Black Caucus as opposed to five in 1965. Despite our progress, Afrikan Americans have yet to achieve full equality in our democracy, and discrimination against minority voters still exists.

Economic and Social Disparities

When we understand that policy decisions foster economic and social disparities in our country, we should also realize that policy is the key to creating more equitable regions throughout the country for all Americans, particularly low-income people of color.

Ultimately, we need a new generation of policies guided by the belief that those closest to the nation's challenges are central to the search for solutions. And statistics indicate that children of color will be vital in fulfilling that need.

It's also highly suggested that the prosperity of our nation will be increasingly dependent on the knowledge and contributions of students/children of color. No matter how we choose to see or look at it, all avenues and roads of approach lead us back to the children, our children, Black children. Therefore, we must teach them early on how to be critical thinkers.

They must know how to reason logically and statistically, avoid fallacies and biases, and be acutely aware of human fallibility, most notably their own. The more we cultivate this mindset, the more we will flourish. As we prepare for the impending challenges, we must also acknowledge that the stakes are incredibly high, particularly for our children for generations to come.

Restoring Protections

After living in Georgia for over 35 years, I can say with certainty that the Georgia of 2022 is not the Georgia of 1965. However, the continued persistence of racially polarized voting is still overtly apparent in Georgia, as it is in many other states and communities across the country.

"Alarming or not," studies show that the levels of political bigotry today surpass racial bigotry. Because we have been so hardwired with intractable political bias, it has become much easier to manipulate voters. The studies also suggest that the levels of bias are so strong that it influences every aspect of life, from where we live to whom we befriend.

The John Lewis Voting Rights Advancement Act (VRAA) is at the center of the Senate battle. The bill would modernize and revitalize the Voting Rights Act of 1965, strengthening legal protections against discriminatory voting policies and practices.

The John Lewis, Voting Rights Advancement Act, responds to current conditions in voting today by restoring the full protections of the original, bipartisan Voting Rights Act of 1965, which was last reauthorized by Congress in 2006 but gutted by the Supreme Court in 2013.

The John Lewis, Voting Rights Advancement Act, also establishes a targeted process for reviewing voting changes in jurisdictions nationwide, focused on measures that have historically been used to discriminate against voters.

The House of Representatives passed an omnibus voting bill that included the John R. Lewis Voting Rights Advancement Act to restore and revitalize the Voting Rights Act of 1965 (VRA). The bill is now before the Senate, and despite bipartisan support, it faces an uncertain future due to the filibuster.

The VRA of 1965 was the most successful civil rights legislation in our country's history until the Supreme Court gutted the law in Shelby County v. Holder in 2013. The court further weakened the law's protections against voting discrimination in Brnovich v. Democratic National Committee in 2022.

This gutting severely weakened the federal government's oversight of discriminatory voting practices. Since the Supreme Court's decision, states and localities have brazenly pushed forward discriminatory changes to voting practices.

The changes include but are not limited to changing district boundaries to disadvantage select voters, instituting more voter identification laws, and changing polling locations with little notice. These laws especially disenfranchise people of color, the elderly, low-income people, transgender people, and people with disabilities.

Voters are more vulnerable to discrimination now than at any time since the Voting Rights Act was signed into law more than fifty years ago. Our nation faces a wave of voting restrictions and redistricting abuses, often targeting communities of color. We need a full-strength Voting Rights Act to prevent this type of suppression.

Moreover, Republicans in the Senate and their allies oppose it. We are now in the midst of a crisis.

The Plot Thickens

Ironically, America stands as a symbol of hope for people in oppressed countries globally because we are perceived as a nation striving to live up to the spirit of one of the most revolutionary documents in the world, the Constitution.

However, America's greatest threat is the proposed actions and results contrary to what the country stands for, all in an effort to systematically arrange personal beliefs as law, grossly undermining our political, ethical, and moral foundation.

In every national election, voters have faced efforts to reduce turnout, particularly Afrikan Americans and other minorities. We must also understand that while the violence of the post-Civil War voter suppression tactics, poll taxes, and the Jim Crow era literacy tests may be behind us, more subtle and creative tactics have taken their place.

More to the point, Republican politicians have developed an even more divisive, exclusive, and oppressive campaign to keep these groups from the polls by using tactics that range from passing restrictive laws to radical gerrymandering, all done deliberately and overtly.

Gerrymandering is the practice of dividing or arranging a territorial unit into election districts in a way that gives one political party an unfair advantage in elections. Results are achieved by manipulating the boundaries of an electoral constituency.

This practice has been a thorn in the side of democracy for centuries, and with the new round of restrictions, it's a bigger threat now than ever before. Since 2010 Republicans have led the charge for voter restrictions, and a majority of Republican states have tightened voting restrictions in ways that make it harder for minorities to vote.

The ridiculously inadequate reason politicians (Republicans) give the public for enacting these restrictive measures is to prevent voter fraud. Yet, "virtually all the significant scholarship on voter impersonation fraud has concluded that it is rare and nowhere near the numbers necessary to affect any election."

The real reason why some people, mainly Republicans, try to keep them (the poor, minorities, and the young) from the polls is that these groups tend to vote for Democratic candidates, and by making it harder for them to vote, Republicans can tilt elections in their favor.

We must be mindful that being a member of a democracy takes work, because democracy is a machine that often requires maintenance. And our votes provide that necessary routine maintenance.

Moreover, voting is the most effective way to ask, Are you hearing us? Participating in elections is also one of the key freedoms of American life. So, exercising your right to vote is crucial no matter what you believe or who you support.

We must acknowledge and teach our children that voting is still one of our most powerful tools for change. A single vote can decide an election, and a single voter can lead to sweeping social change.

Ultimately, we shouldn't encourage our children to vote out of guilt based on civic duty. We must teach them the wisdom of voting based on economic self-interest to give them, their families, and their communities more opportunities.

Shem Hotep (I go in peace)

Chapter 7
Our Children's Mental Health

Mental Health Crisis

"Mental health is the springboard of thinking and communication skills, learning, emotional growth, resilience, and self-esteem."

Our children's mental health is in crisis and now is the time to demand change with our voices and actions. We must also understand that our obligation to act is not just medical; it's moral. Mental health encompasses our emotional, psychological, and social well-being; it is essential to overall health.

It affects every aspect of our lives: how we feel about ourselves and the world, solve problems, cope with stress, overcome challenges, build relationships, and connect with others. Moreover, our children's and youth's mental health will also determine their performance in school, at work, and throughout life.

For those who have been critically looking, we are now witnessing soaring rates of mental health challenges among our children, adolescents, and their families resulting from the COVID-19 pandemic, exacerbating the systemic challenges that existed before the pandemic.

Since the pandemic began, rates of psychological distress among our children have increased. Mental illness and the demand for psychological services are at all-time highs. Unfortunately, the pandemic has struck at the safety and stability of our children and their families across the country, resulting in enormous adversity and disruption.

Notably, for Black Americans, this worsening crisis in child and adolescent mental health is inextricably tied to the stress brought on by COVID-19 and the ongoing struggle for racial justice, which has also exacerbated systemic trends observed before COVID-19.

The inequities that result from systemic racism have contributed to the disproportionate impact on children from communities of color. Therefore, systemic change is necessary in revitalizing communities of color. Change can't come soon enough for a generation of children facing unprecedented pressures and stressors.

The Declaration of a National Emergency

The American Academy of Pediatrics (AAP), the American Academy of Child and Adolescent Psychiatry (AACAP), and the Children's Hospital Association (CHA) have joined together and declared a National State of Emergency in Children's Mental Health.

Over 140,000 children in the United States lost a primary and/or secondary caregiver, resulting from the COVID-19 pandemic, with youth of color disproportionately impacted. We are now seeing our children with soaring rates of depression, anxiety, trauma, loneliness, and suicidality that will have lasting impacts on them, their families, and their communities.

The declaration is designed to identify strategies to meet these challenges through innovation and action, using state, local, and national approaches to improve the access to and quality of care across the continuum of mental health promotion, prevention, and treatment.

AAP, AACAP, and CHA have declared that the challenges facing children and adolescents are so widespread that we call on policymakers at all levels of government and advocates for children and adolescents to join us in this declaration and advocate for the following:

- Increase federal funding dedicated to ensuring all families and children, from infancy through adolescence, can access evidence-based mental health screening, diagnosis, and treatment to appropriately address their mental health needs, with particular emphasis on meeting the needs of under-resourced populations.

- Address regulatory challenges and improve access to technology to ensure continued availability of telemedicine to provide mental health care to all populations.

- Increase implementation and sustainable funding of effective models of school-based mental health care, including clinical strategies and models for payment.

- Accelerate the adoption of effective and financially sustainable models of integrated mental health care in primary care pediatrics, including clinical strategies and models for payment.

- Strengthen emerging efforts to reduce the risk of suicide in children and adolescents through prevention programs in schools, primary care, and community settings.

- Address the ongoing challenges of the acute care needs of children and adolescents, including shortage of beds and emergency room boarding, by expanding access to step-down programs from inpatient units, short-stay stabilization units, and community-based response teams.

- Fully fund comprehensive, community-based systems of care that connect families in need of behavioral health services and support for their child with evidence-based interventions in their home, community, or school.

- Promote and pay for trauma-informed care services that support relational health and family resilience.

- Accelerate strategies to address longstanding workforce challenges in child mental health, including innovative training programs, loan repayment, and intensified efforts to recruit underrepresented populations into mental health professions, as well as attention to the impact the public health crisis has had on the well-being of health professionals.

- Advance policies that ensure compliance with and enforcement of mental health parity laws.

The Advisory

A Surgeon General's Advisory is a public statement that calls the American people's attention to an urgent public health issue and provides recommendations for how it should be addressed. Advisories are reserved for significant public health challenges that need the nation's immediate awareness and action.

The U.S. Surgeon General's Advisory (Protecting Youth Mental Health), issued in 2021, not only gives the problematic background regarding the mental health of our children, it offers recommendations for supporting their mental health and overall well-being.

Further, the advisory includes essential recommendations for the institutions surrounding our children that shape their day-to-day lives. These institutions include but are not limited to schools, community organizations, health care systems, technology companies, media, funders and foundations, employers, and government.

Children of color, notably Black Children, were disproportionately impacted far before the COVID-19 pandemic due to systemic challenges that severely undermine the safe and supportive environments our children need and deserve.

However, our children have experienced other challenges during the pandemic that may have affected their mental and emotional well-being. Particularly our young Black boys, as they see and interpret the stained fabric of our nation, wondering where they fit in.

Our children have experienced the nation's reckoning over the deaths of Black Americans at the hands of white police officers, including the tragic murder of George Floyd. Our youth have observed COVID-related violence against Asian Americans, gun violence, an increasingly polarized political dialogue, growing concerns regarding climate change, and emotionally charged misinformation.

Pandemic-related measures reduced in-person interaction among children, friends, social support, and professionals such as teachers, school counselors, pediatricians, and child welfare workers. This dynamic made it harder to recognize signs of child abuse, mental health concerns, and other challenges.

Although the pandemic's long-term impact on our children and young people is not fully understood, there is still cause for optimism. We have an unprecedented opportunity as a country to rebuild in a way that refocuses our identity and common values, puts people first, and strengthens our connection to each other.

What We Can Do

There is much to be done, and each of us has a role to play. Supporting the mental health of our children and young people will require a whole-of-society effect. To mitigate the pandemic's mental health impact, we must address long-standing challenges, strengthen the resilience of our youth, and avidly support their families and communities.

In protecting our children's mental health, here is some of what we must do:

- Recognize that mental health is essential to overall health, which must be reflected in how we communicate about and prioritize mental health.

- Empower youth and their families to recognize, manage, and learn from difficult emotions. Youth and families should know that asking for help is a sign of strength.

- Ensure that every child has access to high-quality, affordable, and culturally competent mental health care.

- Support the mental health of children and youth in education, community, and childcare settings. To achieve this, we must also expand and support the early childhood and educational workforce.

- Address the economic and social barriers that contribute to poor mental health for young people, families, and caregivers.

- Increase timely data collection and research to rapidly identify and respond to youth mental health needs. The country needs an integrated, real-time data infrastructure for understanding youth mental health trends.

What Our Children Can Do

Since many of the challenges young people face are outside of their control, we need a whole-of-society effort to support our children's mental health and well-being from birth to adulthood.

There are crucial steps children and young people themselves can take to protect, improve, and advocate for their mental health and that of their family, friends, and neighbors.

- Remember that mental health challenges are real, common, and treatable.

- Ask for help. Find trusted adults, friends, or family members to discuss stressful situations. Reaching out to others can be challenging and takes courage, but it's worth the effort and reminds us we are not alone.

- Invest in healthy relationships. Social connection is a powerful buffer to stress and a source of well-being.

- Find ways to serve. Service is a powerful antidote to isolation, and it reminds our children that they have value to add to the world.

- Learn and practice techniques to manage stress and other difficult emotions. Recognize emotional challenges and come up with strategies to manage those emotions.

- Take care of your body and mind. Stick to a schedule, eat well, stay physically active, get quality rest, stay hydrated, and spend time outside.

- Be intentional about using social media, video games, and other technologies. How much time are you spending online? Is it taking away from healthy offline activities, like exercising, seeing friends, reading, and sleeping?

- Be a source of support for others.

What Educators, School Staff, and School Districts Can Do

Mental health challenges can reveal themselves in various ways at school. Experiences our children have at school significantly impact their mental health. They can learn new knowledge and skills at school, develop close relationships with peers and supportive adults, and find a sense purpose, fulfillment, and belonging.

Here are a few essential recommendations for how schools, educators, and staff can support the mental health of all students:

- Create positive, safe, and affirming school environments.

- Expand social and emotional learning programs and other evidence-based approaches that promote healthy development.

- Learn how to recognize signs of mental and physical health change among students, including trauma and behavior changes. Take appropriate action when needed.

- Provide a continuum of support to meet student mental health needs, including evidence-based prevention practice and trauma-informed mental health care.

- Expand the school-based mental health workforce.

- Support the mental health of all school personnel.

- Promote enrolling and retaining eligible children in Medicaid, CHIP, or a Marketplace plan so that children have health coverage that includes behavioral health services.

- Protect and prioritize students with higher needs and those at higher risk of mental health challenges.

What Health Care Organizations and Health Professionals Can Do

Our healthcare system today is not set up to optimally support our children and youth's mental health and well-being. In addition to changing government policy, we must reimagine how healthcare organizations and health professionals prevent, identify, and address mental health challenges.

Here are some steps healthcare organizations and health professionals can take:

- Recognize that the best treatment is the prevention of mental health challenges. Implement trauma-informed care (TIC) principles and other prevention strategies to improve care for all youth, especially those with a history of adversity.

- Routinely screen children for mental health challenges and risk factors, including adverse childhood experiences (ACEs). Screening can be done in primary care, schools, emergency departments, and other settings.

- Identify and address the mental health needs of parents, caregivers, and other family members.

- Combine the efforts of clinical staff with those of trusted community partners and child-serving systems.

- Build multidisciplinary teams to implement services tailored to the needs of children and their families. Additionally, support the well-being of mental health workers and community leaders, building their capacity to support youth and their families.

What Media Organizations, Entertainment Companies, and Journalists Can Do

Media organizations, entertainment companies, and journalists can profoundly impact young people. In some cases, this impact can be positive. On the other hand, false, misleading, or exaggerated media narratives can perpetuate misconceptions and stigma against people with mental health issues. In addition, media coverage of traumatic events can contribute to psychological distress.

- Recognize the impact media coverage of adverse events can have on the public's mental health. The solution isn't to hide or downplay negative news but to avoid misleading consumers and be more attentive to how stories are framed.

- Being fact-based in reporting and avoiding language that shocks, provokes, or creates a sense of panic. Being more cautious about showing distressing content, particularly graphic images or video, without context or warnings for viewers.

- Giving audiences context, including highlighting uncertainties and conflicting reports. When discussing preliminary research—such as papers that have not yet been peer-reviewed—outlets should be forthright about the incomplete nature of the findings, get independent experts to weigh in, and identify areas of uncertainty.

- Offering the public ways to make a positive difference and including positive messages and stories of hope and healing.

- Normalize stories about mental health and mental illness across all forms of media, taking care to avoid harmful stereotypes, promote scientifically accurate information, and include stories of help, hope, and healing.

- Avoiding harmful stereotypes and demeaning language regarding mental illness. This includes using language that focuses on the person rather than a disease label. Include stories of people seeking help, getting treatment, and successfully recovering.

- Direct consumers to mental health resources (as part of any mental health-related TV episode, movie, news story, podcast, or other media).

- Craft more authentic stories by consulting with subject matter experts and people with personal experience of mental illness or mental health challenges.

What Community Organizations Can Do

Thousands of community organizations are working daily to support the mental health of children and young people. While different groups address different parts of the problem, serve different youth populations, and implement different solutions, all community organizations can keep the following recommendations in mind as they continue their work.

- Educate the public about the importance of mental health, and reduce negative stereotypes, bias, and stigma around mental illness. Community groups can play a crucial role in fostering open dialogue about mental health locally and correcting misconceptions and biases.

- It's particularly important to address misconceptions in populations with an outsized influence over young people, such as families, educators, healthcare professionals, juvenile justice officials, online influencers, and the media.

- Implement evidence-based programs that promote healthy development, support children, youth, and their families, and increase their resilience.

- Include youth enrichment programs, mentoring, skill-based parenting, and family relationship approaches, and other efforts that address social determinants of youth health, such as poverty, exposure to trauma, and lack of access to education and health care.

- Ensure that programs rigorously evaluate mental health-related outcomes. For example, track outcomes around anxiety, depression, and suicide as well as upstream risk and protective factors.

- Address the unique mental health needs of at-risk youth, such as racial and ethnic minorities, LGBTQ+ youth, and youth with disabilities. Youth-serving organizations should think intentionally about how and to whom program services are offered

- For example, actively recruit and engage populations who have historically been prevented from equal access to opportunities and may benefit the most from services. Engage with youth to understand what unique barriers prevent them from accessing mental health services.

- Recruit program staff directly from communities being served. Build program staff capacity to recognize personal biases, as well as structural challenges in these communities.

- Elevate the voices of children, young people, and their families. Youth are experts on their own lives, so engaging youth in community-based mental health efforts is important.

- Explore youth advisory councils and other ways to involve young people in all phases of programming from ideation to implementation. Gather feedback to understand what is and isn't working.

What Funders and Foundations Can Do

Philanthropic and other funding organizations play a critical role in supporting our children and young people's mental health across the entire continuum of need. They can also serve as reliable partners to community-based organizations nationwide, and promote and build cross-sector partnerships.

Recommendations for how funding organizations can support youth mental health:

- Create sustained investments in equitable prevention, promotion, and early intervention.

Prioritize interventions that address social and economic factors known to affect children's healthy development and mental health, such as poverty, discrimination, and inequality, among others.

- Incentivize coordination across grantees and foster cross-sector partnerships to maximize reach and bring together a diversity of expertise. The scale and complexity of mental health issues among young people require collaborative approaches.

- Consider leveraging resources across sectors to advance practices, policies, and research that support the mental health of our children, youth, and families. And support grantees in developing and sharing meaningful mental health outcome measures.

- Scale up evidence-based interventions, technologies, and services. Use a structured process to assess an intervention's readiness to scale and support high-quality implementation at a community level.

- Invest in innovative approaches and research on mental health. Develop and test new solutions, including digitally enabled solutions that can reach young people at scale and in underserved communities.

- Elevate and amplify the voices of youth and families in all stages of funding and evaluation. Engage youth from different identities and backgrounds— particularly those that come from vulnerable communities.

Listening to young people is critical to understanding what kind of solutions will work and what communities need to scale successful interventions.

What Employers Can Do

Employers can play an outsized role in supporting the mental health of children and young people. They can directly help younger employees, such as high school students working part-time jobs or young adults starting out in the labor force after high school or college.

Employers can provide affordable health insurance that covers mental health needs. They can also support children and youth indirectly in a way that promotes work-life balance and a positive culture at work to reduce family stress.

Recommendations for how employers can support the mental health of young people:

- Provide access to comprehensive, affordable, and age-appropriate mental health care for all employees and their families, including dependent children.

Research shows that parental mental health challenges not only impact their productivity in the workplace, but can also affect the mental health of their children.

- Employers should offer health insurance plans that include no or low out-of-pocket costs for mental health services and a robust network of high-quality mental health care providers.
- Implement policies that address underlying drivers of employee mental health challenges, including both home and workplace stressors.

Employers should offer paid family leave and sick leave where feasible. Ensure employees are aware of and can easily make use of these benefits.

Create a workplace culture that affirms the importance of the mental health and well-being of all employees and their families.

Create space for employees to speak up about their feeling and encourage company leaders to serve as role models for discussing mental health and modeling healthy behaviors.

Solicit ideas from employees about how to support their mental health and well-being as well as that of their children and families. Adopt clear messaging that promotes mental health awareness and addresses common misconceptions.

Provide managers and supervisors with training to help recognize negative mental health symptoms in themselves and colleagues and encourage employees to seek help.

Regularly assess employees' sense of well-being within the workplace. Tools such as employee surveys can help employers understand the well-being of employees across demographic groups (e.g., gender, race, sexual orientation) to identify opportunities for improvement.

Employers should assess the well-being of young adults just starting out in the workforce, as well as of parents with young children.

What Federal, State, Local, and Tribal Governments Can Do

Note: For actions taken by the Biden Administration from January to October 2021 to support youth mental health, see Fact Sheet: Improving Access and Care for Youth Mental Health and Substance Use Conditions.

Ultimately, youth mental health challenges cannot be addressed solely by the efforts of youth, their families, local communities, and private organizations. Federal, state, local, and tribal governments all have a role to play.

While the below recommendations are not comprehensive, their implementation would mark an enormous step forward in supporting youth and their families:

- Address the economic and social barriers that contribute to poor mental health for young people, families, and caregivers.

- Priorities should include reducing child poverty and ensuring access to quality childcare, early childhood services, education, healthy food, affordable health care, stable housing, and safe neighborhoods with amenities such as parks and playgrounds.

Recent federal investments in child poverty reduction, safe school reopening, and other pandemic-related measures represent historic progress on this front. Still, additional investments are needed at all levels of government.

- Emphasis should be placed on preventing adverse childhood experiences (ACEs), which are substantial risk factors for mental health challenges.

- Take action to ensure safe experiences online for children and young people. Opportunities include but are not limited to increasing investment in research on the role of social media and technology in youth mental health and educating consumers about potential mental health risks online.

Ultimately requiring companies to be more transparent with researchers and the public (e.g., disclosing meaningful data for research purposes, enabling systemic auditing of social media algorithms) and developing safety standards for online services.

For instance, the United Kingdom's Age-appropriate design code has led companies, including Instagram, TikTok, and YouTube, to announce product changes to protect their users' safety, rights, and privacy.

- In addition, the Australian government's Safety by Design initiatives has resulted in a set of principles for user safety, tools for companies to assess their safety practices, resources for investors and financial entities to manage online safety risks, and a pilot program with universities to embed Safety by Design materials into curricula.

- Ensure all children and youth have comprehensive and affordable coverage for mental health care. Opportunities include strengthening public and private insurance coverage for children and young adults.

- Ensuring adequate payment for pediatric mental health services, investing in innovative payment models for integrated and team-based care, increasing the participation of mental health professionals in insurance networks, and ensuring compliance with mental health parity laws are crucial.

- Support integration of screening and treatment into primary care. For example, continue expanding Pediatric Mental Health Care Access programs, which give primary care providers teleconsultations, training, technical assistance, and care coordination to support diagnosis, treatment, and referral for children with mental health and substance use needs.

- Expanding screening for ACEs is also critical. For instance, California recently enacted a law that will significantly expand coverage for ACEs screening.

This recent law will ensure that all middle and high school students learn about mental health in health education classes. In New Jersey, a recent program will provide funding for school districts to screen students for depression.

- Provide resources and technical assistance to strengthen school-based mental health programs.

- Opportunities include improving education about mental health, increasing screening of students for mental health concerns, investing in additional staff to support student mental health needs, improving care coordination, and financing school-based mental health services.

- The American Rescue Plan's Elementary and Secondary School Emergency Relief funds can be used for these purposes, along with Project AWARE (Advancing Wellness and Resilience in Education) program funds, which provide support for state, local, and tribal governments.

- Support building school-provider partnerships and coordinating resources to support prevention, screening, early intervention, and mental health treatment for youth in school-based settings are crucial.

- Invest in prevention programs, such as evidence-based social and emotional learning.

Opportunities include implementing developmentally appropriate social emotional learning standards programs.

- Supporting professional development for educators and providing funding for teachers and school leaders to work with families to support student health needs.

- Expand the use of telehealth for mental health challenges. Opportunities include addressing regulatory barriers, ensuring appropriate payment, and expanding broadband access.

For instance, Colorado recently established the "I Matter" program, offering young people three free behavioral health sessions, primarily via telehealth.

- Expand and support the mental health workforce. Opportunities include investing in training and hiring individuals from a broader set of disciplines, accelerating training and loan repayment initiatives, supporting health workers' mental health and well-being and recruiting a diverse workforce that reflects local communities.

In the school setting, governments should invest in building a pipeline of school counselors, nurses, social workers, and school psychologists.

- Expand and strengthen suicide prevention and mental health crisis services. Opportunities include providing flexible funding to fund crisis care needs and increasing access to intensive outpatient and other "step-down" programs.
- Supporting access to trauma-informed services for traumatized children, implementing the 988 mental health crisis and suicide prevention hotline, and promoting public awareness of crisis hotlines and other resources.

Governments should also collaborate with the private sector and local communities to reduce access to firearms and other lethal means of suicide and promote best practices such as safe storage.

- Improve coordination across all levels of government to address youth mental health needs. One example is to ensure households eligible for social services and supports are receiving the.

- For instance, states can align renewal processes across Medicaid and the Supplemental Nutrition Assistance Program (SNAP), use data from SNAP files to complete Medicaid renewal, and allow qualified entities like schools to make presumptive eligibility determinations. Support continued reduction in biases, discrimination, and stigma related to mental health. Example opportunities include enforcing laws that support the needs of at-risk youth (e.g., students with disabilities).

- Identifying and improving policies and programs that inappropriately target or harm youth with mental health needs and conducting targeted education campaigns to address stigma, promote new cultural norms, and increase safety and trust in local communities.

- Support the mental health needs of youth involved in the juvenile justice system. Example opportunities include investing in alternatives to incarceration (e.g., school, probation, and police-based diversion models for youth with mental health needs).

Expanding mental health training for staff, supporting high-quality and trauma-informed mental health care inside these systems, and improving coordination across different youth-serving agencies are essential for our children and youth in need.

- Support the mental health needs of youth involved in the child welfare system. Example opportunities include expanding family-centered mental health services to prevent unnecessary entry and increase reunification.

- Ensuring youth and caregivers are informed about medications; investing in peer support services; providing mental health services before, during, and after new placements and when emancipating from foster care.

- Ensuring youth have access to mental health services in community settings whenever possible and avoiding unnecessary placements in non-family settings. Coordination should be improved across different youth-serving agencies.

Where Additional Research is Needed

Despite the evidence that millions of young people are suffering and in crisis, there is still a lot we don't know. Recommendations for research questions and studies that should be prioritized to better understand and address youth mental health needs:

Improve mental health data collection and integration to understand youth mental health needs, trends, services, and evidence-based interventions.

Today, data on youth mental health are collected and analyzed by multiple agencies and often take months or years to be released.

The federal government should strengthen research and data integration across governments, health systems, and community organizations to ensure regular surveillance of national mental health trends across the age continuum.

Data should be able to be disaggregated to enable analysis of trends (by age, gender, race, ethnicity, disability status and type, sexual orientation, socioeconomic background, family characteristics, insurance status, etc.)

Foster public-private research partnerships. For example, academic partners, community-based organizations, technology companies, healthcare companies, and others can partner to conduct novel studies.

Using nontraditional data sources to understand needs better, track outcomes, and evaluate risk and protective factors for youth mental health. Increase investments in basic, clinical, and health services research to identify treatment targets for mental health conditions and develop innovative, scalable therapies. Prioritize data and research with at-risk youth populations, such as racial, ethnic, and sexual and gender minority youth, individuals from lower socioeconomic backgrounds, youth with disabilities, youth involved in the juvenile justice system, and other groups.

Researchers and research sponsors should ensure that these populations are represented in basic, translational, effective, and services research studies.

This method will help improve understanding of disparities in risk and trajectories for mental illnesses, responsiveness to interventions, and access to and engagement with quality mental health services.

Advance dissemination and implementation science to scale up and improve compliance with evidence-based mental health practices in systems that serve children, youth, and their families.

Appropriate funding agencies can prioritize demonstration projects of effective evidence-based interventions in and across schools or other systems (e.g., primary care offices, clinics, treatment facilities, family services, child welfare settings, and juvenile justice settings).

Translate findings into actionable policy proposals and disseminate them effectively to improve the adoption of the best practices.

Conduct research to expand understanding of social media and digital technology's impact on youth mental health and identify opportunities for intervention.

For example, explore the impact of frequent exposure to social comparisons, hateful speech, and graphic content on children and youth and which groups are most and least affected.

Also, identify opportunities for families to engage with youth around social media as a means of connection and offer guidance in handling difficult interactions and content.

Explore how pre-existing mental health status and environmental conditions in young people's lives inform how they engage with and experience content online and empower young people with effective strategies to actively manage their online experiences.

Conclusion

As we continue learning and navigating the lessons of the COVID-19 pandemic and start recovering and rebuilding, we have an opportunity to demand a more comprehensive, more fulfilling, and more conclusive vision of what constitutes public health.

As I finish this chapter, I'm reminded of a question my father would occasionally ask me, notable after a persuasive conversation. He would say, "Well, son, you can surely talk the talk, but can you walk the walk?" It is now time for our Nation to "Walk the Walk."

Only when we do will we be able to protect, strengthen, and support the health and safety of all our children, adolescents, and young adults—and ensure they have a platform to thrive.

Hotep (Peace)

[1] This chapter includes excerpts and recommendations from the AAP-AACAP-CHA Declaration of a National Emergency in Child and Adolescent Mental Health and The U.S. Surgeon General's Advisory: Protecting Youth Mental Health. For further information, see the bibliography.

Chapter 8
In Living Color

Sadly, true knowledge often gives way to distorted perceptions of reality that are often accepted as legitimate scholarship. Therefore, I will provide an unparalleled perception in living color.

The Objective

I am not a racist by any means; I am a Black man, a Black husband, a Black father and most importantly, a child of the "Most High" with a distinctive past that history refuses to acknowledge. I am of Afrikan descent, as we all are to some degree or another. However, I can accept or admit the existence or truth of that irrefutable fact.

Because of history's profound disdain for Afrikan/ Black people, I wanted my children to know and understand that, in reality, there is only one race, " the human race," which has been irrefutably proven to have originated in Africa.

Exposing my children to our compelling story was to bring truth to their reality and build character by showing and teaching them the distinctive nature of our Afrikan origin by acknowledging the established precedents of our spiritual, historical, and cultural significance as Black people.

My ultimate objective is to inform and prepare all children, particularly children of color, for a world that is changing and not changing.

Writing

My writing is not intended to be offensive to anyone by any means. However, my intent is not to impress you but to inform you and continue bringing forth new scholarship to challenge Western civilization at its flawed foundation.

I am truly grateful and humbled to have been exposed to and guided through years of extensive research and exploratory travels to further document and substantiate my writing. I have also been blessed and highly favored regarding my life experiences and intimacies along the way. And for that, I am eternally grateful.

Writing has become my labor of love allowing me to willingly take the necessary risks associated with the indoctrination of an inherent ideology (The Afrikan Legacy/Our Story). A story that I've internalized, taught, and implemented. It has also allowed me to articulate who I am, where I come from, and where I still must go.

Like many of my Ancestors and elders who've come before me, I too, feel obligated to reveal fundamental truths concerning the contributions of the Afrikan continent to civilization, given the things that I've seen, touched, and experienced.

The information I've researched and written about is extremely vital to our Afrikan/Black community, particularly at this time throughout the globe. Therefore, I will continue to reiterate that talking about racism, oppression, and their effect on people of color, is not an attempt to guilt or shame anyone.

It is a conscious effort to spread awareness in an attempt to identify and adequately address the systemic problems that Afrikan/Black Americans face. For some, these efforts will be more challenging to grasp than for others. However, we must understand that evoking change is a long process, but learning more about systemic racism and oppression is a necessary first step for all Americans.

Therefore, providing information and knowledge free from error in accordance with fact and truth is vital. My first book, _From Plight to Promise,_ provides a foundation based on valuable insight and firsthand knowledge through eyewitness accounts as opposed to subjective interpretation.

From Plight to Promise is interest-evoking, conviction-inspiring, and a powerfully irrefutable read. It will introduce to some and enhance for others the knowledge and understanding of a fundamental culture which was designed to give meaning to reality.

Our Children and the entire world can benefit by knowing and understanding our amazing story. _From Plight to Promise_ compellingly tells that story, acknowledging that our unique experience, with its many triumphs and tragedies, is still the embodiment of totality.

From Plight to Promise is intended for all people, because it exposes the variable and invariable nature of life and circumstances, but it also provides the necessary wisdom, knowledge, and understanding to address those often uninvited circumstances.

Memory Lane

As I begin writing today, while thinking about our children, their future, and the future of our nation, I'm reminded of the opening lines of the Declaration of Independence.

"We hold these truths to be self-evident that all men are created equal, that they are endowed by their Creator with certain unalienable Rights, that among these are Life, Liberty, and the pursuit of Happiness."

As my mind continues to stroll down memory lane, I am also reminded of the opening line of the Constitution and the final words of the Pledge of Allegiance:

"We the people of the United States, in Order to form a more perfect Union, establish Justice, ensure domestic Tranquility, provide for the common defense, promote the general Welfare, and secure the Blessing of Liberty, to ourselves and *our Posterity do ordain and establish this Constitution for the United States of America."*

And the final words of the Pledge of Allegiance are *"liberty and justice for all."* These words represent a sacred oath, committing ourselves to establish a society where all are free, treated with equal justice, and given equal opportunity to experience tranquility and happiness. Further, the words of America's founders placed its citizens in a contract with one another to establish unity, tranquility, and justice to promote the welfare of all.

Without question, the founding Fathers defined America clearly, with powerful words that cannot be misunderstood. Words that are essential to our society, and if these words cease to have meaning, America will likely have an unfortunate and inescapable outcome.

Ironically, the insightful words of Frederick Douglass also come to mind. In his West India Emancipation speech on August 4, 1857, he stated with extreme certainty, *"If there is no struggle, there is no progress. Power concedes nothing without a demand. It never did, and it never will."*

These words are as insightful today as they were in 1857 due to the perpetuation of oppression through systemic racism. Let us also be mindful that the existence of racism in America is a quantifiable fact.

And to add insult to injury, the complex interactions of large-scale societal systems, practices, ideologies, and programs that produce and perpetuate inequities for racial minorities have become a societal norm.

The State of Black America Today:

Today's America is a fractured society, sharply divided along the lines of race, gender, political party, economic class, and religion. Additionally, the roots of bias and unfairness still remain a perpetual part of America, more than 240 years after its founding document declared that *all men are created equal.*

There is a need for a new direction and narratives to guide us through the twenty-first century and beyond. This consensus is based on what must still be done to ensure that our journey continues to move forward purposefully for all people/children of color in our nation.

That's not to say that we must discard everything that has helped us reach this point. However, we should not be so entangled in tradition that we are unable to rationally evaluate what is still working for us and what's not. Change is imminent!

I am confident that I am only one of many moved and inspired by the 85-year-old Harry Belafonte at the 2013 NAACP Image Awards. He was receiving an award for his nearly 60 years of civil rights activism, and his speech was both inspiring and sobering.

He exclaimed, *"In the gun game, we are the most hunted, and the river of blood that washes the streets of our nation flows mostly from the bodies of our Black children."* After exclaiming these unfortunate truths to the mostly Black audience, he soberingly asked, "Where is the raised voice of Black America? Why are we mute?"

The generational changing of the guard that has begun is promising and reinvigorating. Activism has always been a survival mechanism for Afrikan Americans, often sparked by actions that trigger emotions. More to the point, Black America has been triggered, and there has been a corresponding resurgence in activism.

A new generation has been moved by the election of Barack Obama, sickened by the murders of George Floyd and others, motivated by the kneeling of Colin Kaepernick, disgusted by the election of Donald Trump, and disillusioned by Republican lawmakers.

We, the people, particularly Black people, should be emotionally triggered by the overall contempt and injustice of a country that has yet to find a way to meet its promise of "liberty and justice for all."

Black Lives Matter

First and foremost, all lives matter and we must understand and respect that. However, any system that deprives a people of its family structure denies the humanity of that people. Further, the developers of such a system defy the Creator of mankind and insults the Creator's creation.

America originated such a system in its slavery scheme introducing a new and different type of slavery. It was designed to destroy all elements of the Black family. History has no equal to match the terrible way in which America intentionally treated and destroyed the Black family. These sad and shameful truths are a vital part of American history.

There is no justification for the brutal, dehumanizing institution of slavery in America.

Racial subordination was codified and enforced by violence, as the nation and its leaders allowed Black people to be burdened, beaten, and marginalized throughout the 20th century.

More to the point, slavery did not end; it evolved. The formal abolition of slavery did nothing to overcome the harmful ideas created to defend it. And systemic/institutional racism is a dreadful but fundamental component of the evolution.

However, far too many(Conservatives/Republicans) seem to conveniently forget that the existence of racism in America is not an opinion; it is a quantifiable fact. Racism is a mindset that is rarely openly articulated but is pervasive throughout our culture. It speaks to and of the institutional or systemic racism hiding in plain sight. It did then, and it does now.

It's almost invisible because it's been around for so long, and people simply refuse to see it. We must understand that racism is not only devastating for people of color, but it is devastating for our entire society. And until we wrestle with the demons that have shaped and framed us, we will not be able to embrace the full measure of our true humanity as citizens in society.

Black Lives Matter has been unfairly scrutinized in an attempt to make it something that it's not. Black Lives Matter is a decentralized political and social movement that seeks to highlight racism, discrimination, and racial inequality experienced by Black people. Its primary concerns are police brutality and racially motivated violence against Black people.

Black Lives Matter (BLM) is also an international activist movement, originating in the African-American community, that campaigns against violence and systemic racism toward Black people. BLM regularly protests police killings of Black people and broader issues of racial profiling, police brutality, and racial inequality in the United States criminal justice system.

In 2013, the movement began with the hashtag #BlackLivesMatter on social media after the acquittal of George Zimmerman in the shooting death of teen Trayvon Martin. Black Lives Matter became nationally recognized for its street demonstrations following the 2014 deaths of two African Americans: Michael Brown, resulting in protests and unrest in Ferguson, Missouri, and Eric Garner in New York City.

The originators of the hashtag and call to action are Alicia Garza, Patrisse Cullors, and Opal Tometi. They expanded their project into a national network of over 30 local chapters between 2014 and 2016. The overall movement is a decentralized network and has no formal hierarchy. Since the Ferguson protests, participants in the movement have demonstrated against the deaths of numerous other African Americans by police actions or while in police custody.

In the summer of 2015, Black Lives Matter activists became involved in the 2016 United States presidential election. There have been many reactions to the Black Lives Matter movement. The U.S. population's perception of Black Lives Matter varies considerably by race.

The phrase "All Lives Matter" sprang up as a response to the Black Lives Matter movement. However, "All Lives Matter" has been criticized for dismissing or misunderstanding the message of Black Lives Matter. Following the shooting of two police officers in Ferguson, the hashtag Blue Lives Matter was created by supporters of the police.

"Woke"

The definition of "woke" changes depending on who you ask. Merriam-Webster Dictionary states that being "woke" politically in the Black community means being informed, educated, and conscious of social injustice and racial inequality. The term "woke" in one of its more contemporary meanings, began gaining popularity at the start of the Black Lives Matter movement in 2014.

The Oxford English Dictionary added "woke" in 2017. The term and its derivatives are commonly used to describe people who are "alert to racial or social discrimination and injustice." Originally slang used by Black Americans, the word became part of the national lexicon in the past few years.

The meaning has already changed, and there is a divide in how the word is perceived, a divide that is both political and generational. However, one of its earliest uses was in a historical recording of the protest song "Scottsboro Boys" by Lead Belly. In that recording, it was used as a term about staying aware of the potential for racist violence as a Black person in America.

Staying "woke," for Black people, is a necessity. We don't choose to be woke; we must be woke to stay alive, to know when we are being exploited in some way. We need to stay woke to know when we are in danger. It is a reflection of the vigilance inherent in Black life.

This process points to something unique about lexical histories: they are born from lived experience and are constantly in flux. Therefore, the evolution of "woke," isn't unusual. And it's not just conservatives on Twitter who are responsible for the changing meaning.

The term has been used by some conservative Republicans as an insult against progressive values. Progressive Black Americans initially coined the term and used it in racial justice movements in the early to mid-1900s to denote an attentiveness to essential issues.

Identity has been at the heart of the so-called culture wars seen across the country, as Democrats and Republicans go head-to-head on issues such as LGBTQ+ rights, racial education in schools, and more.

The word "woke" for many conservative Republicans has come to connote the opposite of what it means. This misunderstanding is often wielded by those who don't recognize how "un-woke" they truly are or are proud of the fact.

We must understand that some people never really grow. They never learn their lesson. They never recognize their mistakes. They never acknowledge their faults. They never admit they were in the wrong. You will never receive an apology from them, and you will never see their behavior change.

A prime example of being "un-woke" and proud of the fact is Florida's Governor Ron DeSantis. In his election night speech, he stated emphatically that "We reject woke ideology and we will never ever surrender to the woke agenda." The pressure against "woke-ness" in Florida has already led to the apparent erasure of race-related content in education.

The content includes but is not limited to, the rejection of an AP African American history course in state high schools and vows from college presidents against having some race-related content that covers "intersectionality", or the idea that systems of oppression should be the primary lens through which teaching and learning are analyzed and improved upon.

This is a classic case of cultural erasure, the process of gradually removing various traditions from society. More specifically, it is the practice in which a dominant culture attempts to negate, suppress, remove, and, in effect, erase the culture of a subordinate culture.

America will never correct its mistakes if teachers are not allowed to teach about them. Ironically many say that history will judge—however, that isn't a compelling argument when some states are making it illegal to teach history.

The powers that be know. And we as a people must come to know and understand that our personal and collective power is greater than racism once we awaken and unify. That is why so much energy is exerted in this society to keep us asleep, disunified, and disempowered.

In Black and White

The existence of racism in America isn't an opinion; it's a quantifiable fact. Racism is a mindset that is rarely openly articulated but is pervasive throughout our culture. It speaks to and of the institutional or systemic racism hiding in plain sight.

It's almost invisible because it's been around for so long, and people simply refuse to see it. Racism is not only devastating for people of color, particularly our children, but it is also devastating for our entire society.

Black history should be important to everyone because it is the history of people who have profoundly impacted world civilization. However, white Americans control over 85% of the country's wealth. Black Americans possess just over 4%, and Latinos only possess 3%. White families, on average, possess ten times more wealth than Black families. WHY?

In America, the dominant group is white; therefore, racism is white racial and cultural prejudice and discrimination by institutional power and authority used to the advantage of whites and the disadvantage of people of color.

Racism and specific racial outcomes result from complex, changing, and often subtle social and institutional dynamics in conjunction with the explicit and intentional prejudices that affect people of color.

Policy decisions foster economic and social disparities in our country. Therefore, policy is the key to creating more equitable regions throughout the country for all Americans, particularly low-income people of color.

Many other nationalities, particularly Europeans, often accuse Black people of playing the race card as if it's something that doesn't exist. The race card is the chilling effects and results of racism in the forms of bigotry, xenophobia, misogyny, and the ultimate fear of white genetic survival.

It is embedded in the system of white supremacy that has been programmed into the minds of our European counterparts. Moreover, this deceptive web of racism advocating racial hatred and promoting social injustice is often put into practice by the unjust exercise of authority and is widely accepted.

That brings us back to our children of color and how the current events and actions will affect them later. In preparing our children for the future, we must grasp where we are now because this is where we, as a people, can establish ourselves as an invaluable part of society. If not, we risk becoming a permanent underclass with decreasing influence.

It is crucial that we instill in our children a respect for education and an understanding of the power associated with the attainment of knowledge. This power will not only allow them to know and understand that they have a role in creating the world they want to live in, but it will also allow them to actively participate in the process.

Let us also be mindful that the continuing development of parents is essential to ensure that they can advocate for and orchestrate the development of their children. We must never forget that education is an investment in the future of not only the child but the entire family.

So, either we contribute to the education of our children today, or our grandchildren will suffer tomorrow.

WHY?

A clear view of history can make us uncomfortable, but that discomfort allows us to learn, grow and harness our collective power to make this nation what it was truly meant to be. The history of this country is rooted in slavery and the relentless perpetuation thereof. Moreover, if you don't understand the source of the problem, how can you solve it?

"The Story: Slavery Evolved. To justify the brutal, dehumanizing institution of slavery in America, its advocates created a myth of racial difference. Stereotypes and false characterizations of Black people were created to defend their permanent enslavement as "most necessary to the well-being of the negro" – an act of kindness that reinforced white supremacy. The formal abolition of slavery did nothing to overcome the harmful ideas created to defend it, so slavery did not end: it evolved.

In the decades that followed, these beliefs in racial hierarchy took new expression in convict leasing, lynching, and other forms of racial terrorism that forced the exodus of millions of Black Americans to the North and West, where the myth of racial difference manifested in urban ghettos and generational poverty.

Racial subordination was codified and enforced by violence in the era of Jim Crow and segregation, as the nation and its leaders allowed Black people to be burdened, beaten, and marginalized throughout the 20th century.

Progress towards civil rights for African Americans was made in the 1960s, but the myth of racial inferiority was not eradicated. Black Americans were vulnerable to a new era of racial bias and abuse of power wielded by our contemporary criminal justice system. Mass incarceration has had devastating consequences for people of color: at the dawn of the 21st century, one in three Black boys are projected to go to jail or prison in his lifetime."

In essence, an elaborate and enduring mythology about the inferiority of Black people was created to legitimize, perpetuate, and defend slavery in America. The mythology of racial difference survived slavery's formal abolition, was violently reinforced in the era of racial terror lynchings, and fueled fierce resistance to the civil rights movement.

Today our criminal justice system is six times more likely to incarcerate Afrikan/Black American men than white men. If this trend continues; statistically, one of every three Black boys born in America today will be imprisoned. This harsh reality is indicative of slavery's dreadful and intended evolution.

Lynching In America

After slavery was formally abolished, lynchings emerged as a vicious tool of racial control to reestablish white supremacy and suppress Black civil rights. More than 4,400 Afrikan/Black Americans were lynched across twenty states between 1877 and 1950.

These lynchings were terrorism, and the effects of racial terror lynchings are still felt today. Racial terror lynchings were violent and public acts of torture that traumatized Black people throughout the country and were largely tolerated by state and federal officials.

Lynchings in the American South were not isolated hate crimes committed by rogue vigilantes; they were targeted racial violence at the core of a systematic campaign of terror perpetuated in furtherance of an unjust social order.

The lynching era left thousands dead; it significantly marginalized Black people in the country's political, economic, and social systems and fueled a massive migration of Black refugees out of the South.

Additionally, lynching - and other forms of racial terrorism - inflicted deep traumatic and psychological wounds on survivors, witnesses, family members, and the entire African American community.

The Legacy Museum: From Enslavement to Mass Incarceration

Along with the critically acclaimed National Memorial for Peace and Justice, the Legacy Museum presents a unique opportunity for visitors to reckon with challenging aspects of our past. And to my surprise, there were far more white American visitors than Afrikan/Black American visitors.

The Legacy Museum provides a comprehensive history of the United States with a focus on the legacy of slavery. The museum offers an immersive experience with cutting-edge technology, world-class art, and critically important scholarship about American history.

Situated on a site in Montgomery, Alabama, where enslaved Black people were forced to labor in bondage, blocks from one of the most prominent slave auction spaces in America, the Museum is steps away from the rail station where tens of thousands of Black people were trafficked during the 19th century.

The museum provides detailed interactive content and compelling narratives from the Transatlantic Slave Trade and its impact on the North and coastal communities across America through the Domestic Slave Trade and Reconstruction.

Lynching codified racial segregation and the emergence of over-incarceration in the 20th century are examined in depth and brought to life through film, images, and first-person narratives. The Transatlantic Slave Trade wing includes more than

200 sculptures and original animated short films narrated by award-winning artists.

Another extraordinary wing of the museum explores the economics of enslavement, the violence of slavery, sexual violence against enslaved Black women, the commodification of people, and the desperate efforts enslaved people made to stay connected to loved ones.

An awe-inspiring exhibit on Reconstruction documents the important 12-year period in American history with a detailed timeline, short films, and first-person narrative accounts.

The expansive content on lynching is housed in a wing that examines the role of media during the era of racial terror violence. The last words of lynching victims dramatize the suffering racial terrorism imposed on entire communities. Facts about the lynching of children help visitors understand the scale of terror and violence many families endured.

An extremely impressive exhibit containing 800 jars of soil collected around the country as part of Equal Justice Initiative's Community Remembrance Project is a unique and powerful display of the growing community response to reckoning with this painful past.

The Jim Crow era and the movement to confront racial segregation are presented with an extensive exploration of the Montgomery Bus Boycott and the work of legendary civil rights activists. The iconography of Jim Crow is dramatically presented in a collection of actual signs and notices collected from around the country.

Equal Justice Initiative also compiled laws and statutes that codified racial apartheid in America for visitors to read and experience. Barriers to voting for Black people are featured as a central component of how equal rights were undermined throughout this era.

I actually took a poll test and experienced how local officials use these arbitrary and humiliating tests to disenfranchise Black people.

The mass incarceration wing features the voices of people who have been wrongly condemned, unfairly sentenced, and unjustly treated in the American legal system. I learned about the plight of children prosecuted as adults, people with mental illness, people experiencing poverty, and those suffering brutal conditions in some of our nation's prisons and jails.

The Reflection Space was stunning, honoring hundreds of people who worked throughout their lives to challenge racial injustice. In a grand space that features music and powerful images, the history of struggle inspires all to reflect on what we can do to make a difference.

The Legacy Museum also includes a world-class art gallery with major works from the most celebrated Black artists in the country. The gallery includes pieces created specifically for the Legacy Museum. Its entire collection is curated in dialogue with the museum's historical narrative while exploring the role of music and dance in understanding our nation's history and the role of the arts.

Without question, the Legacy Museum is an engine for education about the legacy of racial inequality and for the truth and reconciliation that leads to real solutions to contemporary problems.

The National Memorial for Peace and Justice

The National Memorial for Peace and Justice, is the nation's first memorial dedicated to the legacy of enslaved Black people, people terrorized by lynching, African Americans humiliated by racial segregation and Jim Crow, and people of color burdened with contemporary presumptions of guilt and police violence.

The Memorial opened to the public on April 26, 2018. Work on the memorial began in 2010 when Equal Justice Initiative (EJI) staff began investigating thousands of racial terror lynchings in the American South, many of which had never been documented.

EJI was interested not only in lynching incidents but in understanding the terror and trauma this sanctioned violence against the Black community created. Six million Black people fled the South as refugees and exiles due to these "racial terror lynchings."

The Memorial for Peace and Justice was conceived to create a sober, meaningful site where people can gather and reflect on America's history of racial inequality. Set on a six-acre site, the memorial uses sculpture, art, and design to contextualize racial terror.

The site includes a memorial square with 800 six-foot cor-ten steel monuments to symbolize thousands of racial terror lynching victims—one for each county in the United States where a racial terror lynching took place. The names of the lynching victims are engraved on the columns.

The memorial is more than a static monument. EJI is hopeful that the National Memorial will inspire communities nationwide to enter an era of truth-telling about racial injustice and their local histories.

The museum and memorial are part of EJI's work to advance truth and reconciliation around race in America and to honestly confront the legacy of slavery, lynching, and segregation. Our nation's history of racial injustice casts a shadow across the American landscape.

EJI Director Bryan Stevenson explains, *"This shadow cannot be lifted until we shine the light of truth on the destructive violence that shaped our nation, traumatized people of color, and compromised our commitment to the rule of law and to equal justice."*

Conclusion

Power, greed, fear, and a total disregard for humanity are "Why." Understanding "Why" requires an engagement and articulation with the material, structural, and ideological mechanisms of white supremacy. Therefore, I can make and articulate on the above statement because I am "Woke" aware and actively attentive to important facts and issues (especially issues of racial and social justice).

There is no question that the roots of bias and unfairness remain a perpetual part of America. The ultimate betrayal is the overall contempt and injustice of a country that has yet to find a way to meet its promise of "liberty and justice for all," which has contributed to Black Americans' unmatched inner strength and sensitivity.

Despite the betrayal, broken promises, and a new era of racial bias and abuse, our children must know and understand that Black Lives Matter. And to heal the deep wounds of our present, we must face the truth of our past.

Afrikan/Black Americans face devastating disparities on nearly every possible level, from health to housing, crime to criminal justice, education to economic parity. However, the time has come for us to shift the conversation from acknowledging the pain and devastation to developing a plan of radical reorientation for the sake of our children.

Only then will Afrikan/ Black American children be able to move toward the days we dream of, when equality, justice, and morality are the norms instead of just an aspiration for the future?

Is America truly the beautiful or the land of the free? Well, it depends on who you ask. However, I can say with extreme certainty that if you think America is the land of the free or a valuable gem, then you should be Black and experience it like them.

"Fools try to ignore facts, but wise men must face facts to remain wise. Fools refuse to change their ways and beliefs, but the mental flexibility of the wise man permits him to keep an open mind and enables him to readjust himself whenever it becomes necessary for a change."

Malcolm X

Now that we know "Why" let us look deep into the windows of ourselves and answer the call to action. Why Not?

Ase (It is so)

Reflections

Black History Month

February is Black History Month. However, it's never too early to begin celebrating and teaching our children about the Black leaders of yesterday and today. For me, Black history is a 24/7, 365-day-a-year occupation assigned to me by the Creator himself. Showing me that identification with one's history and culture is the first step toward gaining or regaining a sense of consciousness.

As we begin exploring the Black scientists, politicians, activists, artists, and more who have left their mark on history, it is necessary to encourage our children's curiosity about the contributions and accomplishments of Black people.

In addition to commemorating achievements from the past, Black History Month is a time to consider how this country can better serve our Black children. Afrikan/Black

Americans have made and will continue to make integral contributions to every aspect of American life, from our cultural fabric to our international stature.

More to the point, we must help our children understand the resiliency of Black women and men by discussing the history of unfair and differential treatment towards Black people due to the color of their skin. Discussing Black people's achievements in their fight for justice and equity encourages empathy and understanding.

It teaches our children how to connect their personal experiences with the experiences of others. Ultimately modeling what it looks like to be a life-long learner. To begin with, playing and learning with our children early on is crucial because children are like sponges when learning about history.

Therefore, we must set aside time to watch documentaries and videos about Black leaders throughout history and then ask our children to draw a picture, write a journal entry, or simply engage in discussion to help show what they learned.

Reading books that celebrate Black culture is essential. Picture books show the joys and challenges children of all races, ethnicities, and cultures can relate to as they learn and grow. Understanding and celebrating diverse cultures begin with exploring and reading books that offer windows into Black lives and culture.

We can also explore Black history through art. The arts in general, and Black art in particular, can help reduce the negative stigma often assigned to Blackness. Allowing our children to see that all Black is beautiful. When looking at art created by Black illustrators, designers, and painters, ask your children:

What stands out to them first and why? What Black History story does this art tell them about or remind them of? Do the people look happy, sad, or anxious? And why? Learning about Black art and artists can help our children resist race-based negativity and help them learn more about Black history.

Questions to ask our children should include but are not limited to:

What makes someone a hero? Who are some Black heroes that you have learned about? Who are the Black heroes who have broken barriers in history and today? What is a role model? What Black role models helped to make the world a better place? How can you be a role model at school or in your neighborhood?

We can celebrate Black history and cultural diversity year-round by introducing our children to books, stories, and art reflecting culture and ethnicities. However, when I think about the achievements of Black youth and the hope they represent for the future, I must consider a few facts:

(1) Black youth made up approximately 17 percent of the U.S. youth population in 2020 but were the victims in more than half (57 percent) of youth homicides.

(2) In 2020, Black youth were 2.3 times more likely than their white peers to be arrested.

(3) In 2019, Black youth were 4.4 times more likely than their white peers to be in residential placement.

In light of those statistics, we must be committed to serving all youth with equity and fairness and effecting juvenile justice system reforms that guarantee impartiality and promote community-based alternatives to youth incarceration.

Combating racial and ethnic disparities also includes strengthening resources available to states, and states must develop and implement plans to identify strategies that work to reduce disparities.

I hope you all will join me in commemorating Black History all year —celebrating our young people's achievements while recommitting ourselves to systems and services to help our children fulfill their dreams and promises.

Quotes and State-by-State Listing of Black History and Civil Rights Museums

Quotes referencing stand-out Black History and Civil Rights Museums

"I just want to do God's will. And He's allowed me to go up to the mountain. And I've looked over. And I've seen the Promised Land. I may not get there with you. But I want you to know tonight that we, as a people, will get to the Promised Land." Martin Luther King Jr. gave his Promised Land speech the night before his murder in 1968.

"Our minds are nurtured, our spirits are touched and inspired, our sense of self is enhanced and validated by Black

museums." LaNesha DeBardelaben, Executive Director at NAAM.

"There remains an inarguable need to create inclusive, accessible, and dynamic spaces where all people can see Black lives and experiences valued and reflected." Cameron Shaw, Deputy Director and Chief Curator at CAAM.

"The American people have this to learn: that where justice is denied, where poverty is enforced, where ignorance prevails, and where any one class is made to feel that society is an organized conspiracy to oppress, rob and degrade them, neither persons nor property will be safe." Frederick Douglass, former slave, abolitionist, and Underground Railroad Agent, 1886.

"Their cause must be our cause too. Because it's not just Negroes, but really it's all of us who must overcome the crippling legacy of bigotry and injustice. And we shall overcome." Former US President Lyndon B. Johnson on the introduction of the 1965 Voting Rights Act.

"Our nation's history of racial injustice casts a shadow across the American landscape. This shadow cannot be lifted until we shine the light of truth on the destructive violence that shaped our nation, traumatized people of color, and compromised our commitment to the rule of law and to equal justice." Bryan Stevenson, Founder, Equal Justice Initiative.

"The history of this country is rooted in slavery. If you don't understand the source of the problem, how can you solve it?" Ibrahima Seck, Director of Research at the Whitney Plantation.

Across the United States, Black history museums are endeavoring to tell the African-American story. From highly funded national institutions to volunteer-aided communal initiatives, museums play a significant role in documenting and remembering historical eras, leaders, and injustices that have shaped the Black experience.

Many well-known museums deal with the lasting legacy of slavery, the cruel, sustained anti-Black system of Jim Crow in the Southern states, and the stories of the Civil Rights Movement. However, spaces are also dedicated to lesser-known heroes, sporting pioneers, legendary musicians, and African-American art and culture.

Our children must know and understand our history and the significance of our struggle because we have a glorious heritage that must be communicated and understood. More specifically, we must always look to the past in order to move to the future.

State-by-State List of Black History and Civil Rights Museums

Alabama

National Voting Rights Museum and Institute, Selma

The Legacy Museum: From Enslavement to Mass Incarceration / The National Memorial for Peace and Justice, Montgomery

Alaska

In the absence of a dedicated Black history museum in Alaska, the University of Alaska's Consortium Library is a good resource, as is this article spotlighting African American history in Anchorage.

Arizona

George Washington Carver Museum, Phoenix.

Arkansas

Mosaic Templars Center, Little Rock.

California

California African American Museum, Los Angeles

Museum of the African Diaspora, Los Angeles

Colorado

Black American West Museum, Denver

Connecticut

Prudence Crandall Museum, Canterbury

Delaware

Mitchell Center for African American Heritage, Wilmington

Florida

African-American Research Library and Cultural Center, Fort Lauderdale

Old Dillard Museum, Fort Lauderdale

The Blanchard House Museum of African-American History & Culture, Punta Gorda

LaVilla Museum, Jacksonville

Georgia

The National Center for Civil and Human Rights, Atlanta

Apex Museum, Atlanta

Hawaii

Obama Hawaiian Africana Museum, Honolulu

Idaho

Idaho Black History Museum, Boise

Illinois

Pullman Porter Museum, Chicago

DuSable Museum of African American History, Chicago

Indiana

Freetown Village, Freetown

Iowa

African American Museum of Iowa, Cedar Rapids

Kansas

The Kansas African American Museum, Wichita

Kentucky

Kentucky Center for African American Heritage, Louisville

Louisiana

Whitney Plantation, Wallace

New Orleans African American Museum, New Orleans

Maine

Abyssinian Meeting House, Portland

Maryland

Reginald F. Lewis Museum, Baltimore

Howard County Center of African American Culture, Columbia

Massachusetts

Museum of African American History, Boston

Michigan

Tuskegee Airmen National Historical Museum, Detroit

The Charles H. Wright Museum of African American History, Detroit

Minnesota

Minnesota African American Heritage Museum & Gallery, Minneapolis

Mississippi

Mississippi Civil Rights Museum and Museum of Mississippi History, Jackson

Missouri

Ozarks Afro-American Heritage Museum, Ash Grove

The Negro Leagues Baseball Museum, Kansas City

Montana

In the absence of a dedicated Black history museum in Montana, the Montana African American Heritage Resources Project provides details on the subject.

Nebraska

Great Plains Black History Museum, Omaha

Nevada

The Walker African American Museum & Research Center on the west side of Las Vegas closed in 2017 due to water damage but plans to reopen.

New Hampshire

Black Heritage Trail of New Hampshire, Portsmouth

New Jersey

Afro-American Historical Society Museum, Jersey City

New Mexico

African American Museum and Cultural Center of New Mexico, Albuquerque

New York

Studio Museum Harlem

African Burial Ground National Monument and Visitor Center, Manhattan

North Carolina

International Civil Rights Center and Museum, Greensboro

Ohio

National Underground Railroad Freedom Center, Cincinnati

The Cleveland African American Museum, Cleveland

Oklahoma

Oklahoma Black Museum & Performing Arts Center, Oklahoma City

Oregon

Oregon Black Pioneers, Salem

Pennsylvania

African American Museum, Philadelphia

Rhode Island

Stages of Freedom, Providence

South Carolina

Old Slave Mart Museum, Charleston

South Dakota

South Dakota African American History Museum, Sioux Falls

Tennessee

National Museum of African American Music, Nashville

National Civil Rights Museum, Memphis

Withers Collection Museum and Gallery, Memphis

Slave Haven Underground Railroad Museum, Memphis

Green McAdoo Cultural Center, Clinton

Texas

The Buffalo Soldiers Museum, Houston

African American Museum of Dallas

Houston Museum of African American Culture

Utah

Utah Black History Museum, Salt Lake City

Vermont

Rokeby Museum, Ferrisburgh

Virginia

Black History Museum & Cultural Center of Virginia, Richmond

Washington State

Northwest African American Museum, Seattle

Washington D.C.

National Museum of African American History and Culture, Washington D.C.

West Virginia

Black Voices Museum, Harpers Ferry

Wisconsin

Wisconsin Black Historical Society/Museum, Milwaukee

Milton House, Milton

Wyoming

The Wyoming State Museum's traveling exhibit on Black homesteaders, Empire: A Community of African-Americans on the Wyoming Plains, tours the state regularly. Check local events calendars for more information.

Reflections of Greatness

As Afrikan/Black Americans, we must look beyond and rise above the image of Afrika and her descendants that Europeans created for us and the entire world. However, let us be mindful that the first civilization recorded in history is that of Afrika.

Therefore, as descendants of Afrika, we must realize that we have a cultural memory that extends deep enough to recapture the cultural wealth that has given us the potential that has made us a great people.

Let us also be mindful that our Afrikan Ancestors gave civilization, the arts, the sciences, and mathematics to the world. These are the people who created and developed agriculture, cosmetics, internal medicine, mortuary science, the calendar, and the world's first democracy.

Our Afrikan Ancestors are the people who created the natural sciences, including but not limited to biology, chemistry, physics, astrology, and astronomy. These achievements are just a portion of their many contributions.

When I think of reflections of greatness regarding Black history and Black people of yesterday and today, many come to mind, but Kemet (Egypt) is the specific place that comes to mind. Kemet is a book of history, one of God's great monumental records.

Kemet was an unadulterated, predominantly Black race of people that were ruled by lines of hereditary rulers consisting of Black kings and queens for thirty dynastic periods, yielding over three thousand years of cultural and historical continuance. Kemet's glorious and precedents setting period spanned from approximately 26,000 B.C.E to 343 B.C.E.

What this means is that the earliest documentation of civilization with regard to organized systems of government, education, medicine, and religion was undoubtedly that of the Ancient Afrikan people.

Our people have a glorious heritage that must be communicated and understood. Therefore, we must always look to the past in order to move to the future.

Models for the Development of Human Potentiality (Yesterday and Today)

(c. 2647 - 2628 B.C.E.) The "Afrikan Multi-Genius" Imhotep (he who comes in peace) was one of the most talented men known to this world. He was worshiped in early Christianity as the prince of peace and described as the "first Christ," a title meaning "the anointed one."

Imhotep was the first physician to stand out in world history, the earliest of which historical details have survived. Reports state that he treated more than 200 diseases. And this great Afrikan knew the circulation of blood 4000 years before Europeans understood the study of blood.

Imhotep's efforts in medicine were so outstanding that he was worshiped as a divine medical entity 2,500 years after his death. The Greeks considered him the divine entity (god) of medicine and recognized him as Asclepius.

Not only was the science of medicine first developed in the Nile Valley, but an analysis of the opening lines of the Hippocratic Oath provides further evidence of its Kemetic roots and the personalities associated with its early development.

Sadly, to this day, doctors take the Hippocratic Oath, never knowing that Hippocrates was not the father of medicine. The great Afrikan, Imhotep, was in fact, the "father of medicine," as well as a leader in architecture, astronomy, religion, and writing.

Imhotep's father (Kanofer) built the first stone building underground, while Imhotep built the first stone building above ground. As chief architect of the King's work, he designed the Step Pyramid, a transition between the mastaba tombs of the earlier kings and the true pyramid form that developed later.

He was one of the greatest sages and authors of proverbial wisdom. His philosophy survived in the "Songs of the Harper." He even became the patron of scribes. Imhotep was also a grand astronomer. He discovered the circumference of the earth of about twenty-five thousand miles by studying the movement of the sun during the summer and winter solstices.

Let us also be mindful that the Western world did not even know that the world was round until 1492 A.C.E. Imhotep knew the world was round approximately 4,000 years earlier. Imhotep was truly the "Afrikan Multi Genius," one of the most talented men known to this world.

I would be remiss if I did not acknowledge the "Afrikan Multi Genius's" counterpart, "The Modern-day Imhotep."

<u>"The Modern-day Imhotep" Dr. Cheikh Anta Diop</u> was the most daring Afrikan cultural-nationalist historian, scientist, and non-apologetic Egyptologist/Kemetologist of the twentieth century. He studied the human race's origins and pre-colonial Afrikan culture. He was Born December 29, 1923, in Senegal, West Afrika.

Dr. Diop's multi-faceted methods reflected his varied background as an " anthropologist, historian, physicist, politician, and philosopher. His scholarship on reclaiming Black civilization produced an immense body of knowledge on ancient Egyptian/Kemetic culture, which has the interesting effect of inverting Western cultural assumptions.

He was a champion of Afrikan history, devoting his life and brilliant intellect to proving the critical role Black Egyptians/Kemetic people played in developing the arts and sciences, dispelling long-held ideas that Afrikans contributed nothing of importance to humanity.

According to Dr. Diop's theory, the ancient Egyptians were Negroes, Ancestors of the Southerners. Equally important, this hypothesis was presented with supporting data. Therefore, historians who evade the legitimacy of Egypt/Kemet are neither modest nor objective nor unruffled; he is ignorant, cowardly, and neurotic.

Ultimately, Dr. Diop argues that if the ancient Egyptians were Negroes, then European civilization is but a derivation of Afrikan achievement. In a word, the Black world is the very initiator of the "Western" civilization flaunted before our eyes today.

Their fundamental attributes and personal initiatives have been and will continue to be instrumental in making and shaping our cultural fabric. They are indicative of who we are and where we come from. Psalms 82:6 tells us: *"You are gods, and all of you are sons of the Most High."*

We are all children of God; the reality is that we are all brilliant, gorgeous, talented, and fabulous. However, our fear hides that reality from us. Therefore, despite what history has and has yet to tell and show our children, we have work to do. That being said, I'm reminded of Marianne Williamson's famous quote:

"Our deepest fear is not that we are inadequate. Our deepest fear is that we are powerful beyond measure. It is our light, not our darkness that most frightens us. We ask ourselves, Who am I to be brilliant, gorgeous, talented, and fabulous? Actually, who are you not to be? You are a child of God. Your playing small does not serve the world. There is nothing enlightened about shrinking so that other people will not feel insecure around you. We are all meant to shine, as children do. We were born to make manifest the glory of God that is within us. It is not just in some of us; it is in everyone and as we let our own light shine, we unconsciously give others permission to do the same. As we are liberated from our own fear, our presence automatically liberates others."

Our Ancestors knew and understood that fear is not our ultimate reality and does not replace or change the truth of who we are. Further, we must teach our children that freedom comes when they learn to do their own thinking and gain the courage to act on their own God-given initiative.

Our children always have been and always will be determining factors in the outcome of our plight. Other prime examples of models for the development of human potentiality are our Black youth of yesterday and today.

The Black Youth of Yesterday and Today

Even before visiting Egypt (Kemet), I was always fascinated with "The Boy King" of Egypt. After seeing his tomb in the Valley of the Kings, I understand why and how it dazzled the world.

The gold shrines, masks, jewelry, and other treasures revealed the exquisite artistry and workmanship of Afrikan artists. The items found in his tomb made the world aware of the "Boy King." It certainly made me aware and somewhat empowered. The Boy King's collection was remarkable.

(C. 1338-1328 B.C.E.) <u>Tutankhamen - King Tut, "The Boy King,"</u> ascended the throne when he was only nine years old. During his reign, Kemet (Egypt) regained its prestige and religious and political control.

He became famous in 1922 when Sheik Abdu Nady showed Howard Carter the young king's burial site in the Valley of the Kings. His tomb was one of the most significant archaeological finds of the century.

Jaylen Smith was sworn in as mayor, on the first day of 2023, in Earle, Arkansas. Jaylen Smith's swearing-in marked a historic first: At the ripe old age of 18, Smith won't just add to the small number of teenage mayors elected across the United States; he will also be the youngest Black mayor in the country's history.

Maxwell Alejandro Frost is an American politician, activist, and musician serving as the U.S. representative for Florida's 10th congressional district since 2023. Previously he was the national organizing director for March for Our Lives. Elected at age 25, Frost is a Democrat.

Hanif Johnson is the youngest Magisterial District Judge in Pennsylvania. At 26, Johnson decided to run for a Dauphin County District Judge position. He won the general election on November 7, 2017, for the Dauphin Magisterial District.

(C.1395 - 1358 B.C.E.) Queen Tiye, "The Lady of the Two Lands," The beautiful Nubian woman, married King Amenhotep III at thirteen and became his constant companion. The king associated her with every act of his reign.

Queen Tiye strongly influenced Kemet's (Egypt's) foreign and domestic policies. Foreign officials corresponded with her because of her influential role in political affairs. She also served as the world's first Secretary of State.

Queen Tiye was the fashion pacesetter of her time. Not only was she a woman of beauty, but one with brains. This educated woman had an extensive library with historical, scientific, and religious texts.

Lily Adeleye made history as the youngest Black CEO to have products on the shelves at Walmart when she landed her first deal in 2021 at just six years old. Lily's enterprising and ambitious endeavors speak to a more significant movement among Black women, the largest growing entrepreneurial group in the county.

They represent 42% of new women-owned businesses—three times the amount of the overall female population—and 36% of all Black-owned employer businesses.

Amanda Gorman is the youngest inaugural poet in U.S. history, as well as an award-winning writer and cum laude graduate of Harvard University. She is an American poet and activist. Her work focuses on issues oppression, feminism, marginalization, race, and the African diaspora. Gorman was the first person to be named National Youth Poet Laureate.

Jasmine Twitty is an American associate judge for the Easley, South Carolina, municipal court. At the time of her appointment to the position, she was the youngest judge ever to be appointed or elected as a municipal court judge in U.S. history at the age of 25.

Alena Analeigh Wicker is a 14-year-old American student who is the youngest Black person to be accepted into medical school in the United States and the second-youngest person to be accepted into medical school overall. She is also the youngest ever to work as an intern at NASA.

<u>Abigail Daniella Phillip</u> is a Harvard University grad and an American journalist who works as a CNN political correspondent and weekend anchor. She previously worked for The Washington Post, ABC News, and Politico.

More to the point, no matter how we look at it or choose to see it, all relevant roads and avenues of approach lead us back to the original source; Mother Afrika, the home of humanity and a people of first.

We must never forget that power comes in knowing. We must also be mindful that the same wisdom, knowledge, and insight our Ancestors had yesterday we have today. Now is the time to truly educate and reindoctrinate our children.

Ase (It is so)

Bibliography

American Academy of Pediatrics. Declaration of a National Emergency in Child and Adolescent Mental Health. 10/19/2021.

Angelou, Maya. *THE BLACK FAMILY PLEDGE*, 2005.

ben-Jochannan, Yosef A.A. *CULTURAL GENOCIDE: in the Black and African Studies Curriculum.* Baltimore: Black Classic Press, 2004.

Browder, Anthony T. *Nile Valley Contribution to Civilization.* Washington, DC: Institute of Karmic Guidance, 1992.

Diop, Cheikh Anta. *THE AFRICAN ORIGIN OF CIVILIZATION: Myth or Reality.* Edited and translated by Mercer Cook. Chicago: Lawrence Hill Books, 1974.

Garvey, Marcus Mosiah. *The Philosophy and Opinions of MARCUS GARVEY: Afrika for the Afrikans.* Connecticut: Martino, 2014.

Head, Raymond J. *From Plight to Promise. Born into the Lie-Resurrected into the truth.* Cheimsford, MA: Nehas Publishing, 2021.

Hatfield, Frederick C. *FITNESS: THE COMPLETE GUIDE.* Santa Barbara: International Sports Sciences Association(ISSA) 1996.

Jabbar, Kareem Abdul and Obstfeld, Raymond. *WRITINGS ON THE WALL.* New York: Liberty Street, 2016.

Khamit-Kush, Indus. *What They Never Told You In History Class.* Chicago: African American Images, 1983.

King, Coretta Scott. *A TESTAMENT OF HOPE: THE ESSENTIAL WRITINGS AND SPEECHES OF MARTIN LUTHER KING, JR.* New York: Harper-Collins, 1986.

Kozol, Jonathan. *THE SHAME OF THE NATION.* New York: Crown Publishers, 2005.

Kwesi, Ashra, and Merira Kwesi. *Afrikan Builders of Civilization: A Pictorial History of Famous Personalities from Ancient Egypt.* Dallas: Kemet Nu Productions, 2005.

Law-Nolte, Dorothy. *Children Learn What They Live.* 19

Ledesma, Maria C. and Calderon, Dolores. *Critical Race Theory in Education: A Review of Past Literature and a Look to the Future.* 2015.

Martin, Roland S. *WHITE FEAR.* Dallas: Nu Vision Media, Inc, 2022.

Simon, Elliott. American Council on Exercise. *PERSONAL TRAINER MANUAL.* San Diego: Cole Publishing,1991.

Smiley, Group, Inc. *THE COVENANT.* Chicago: Third World Press, 2006.

Taylor, Kiara. *The Digital Divide.* Investopedia.com: 2022.

Taylor, Susan. *In the Spirit.* HarperPerennial: 1st Edition, 1994.

The U.S. Surgeon General's Advisory. *PROTECTING YOUTH MENTAL HEALTH.* 2021.

Welsing, Frances Cress. *The Isis Papers: The Keys to the Colors.* New York: CW Publishing, 2004.

Williams, Chancellor. *THE DESTRUCTION OF BLACK CIVILIZATION: Great Issues of a Race from 4500B.C. to 2000 A.D.* 3rd ed. Chicago: Third World Press, 1987.

Williams, Richard. *THEY STOLE IT BUT YOU MUST RETURN IT.* Rochester, New York: HEMA, 1991.

Woodson, Carter G. *THE MIS-EDUCATION OF THE NEGRO.* The Associated Publishers, 1933.

About the Author

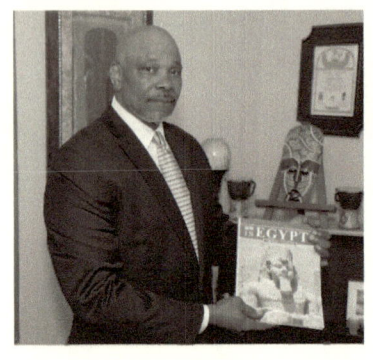

Driven by passion and the need to provide the necessary cultural substance for children, particularly children of color. Raymond is convinced that a legacy of money cannot replace a heritage of dignity.

He avidly studies Afrika because he can't know his history or heritage without her. Without that knowledge, he can't know himself or sufficiently aid our children in knowing who they are, where they come from, and where they still must go.

His first outstanding work, *From Plight to Promise*, provides a foundation based on valuable insight and firsthand knowledge through eyewitness accounts. He expands on that foundation in his second book, entitled *WHY?*

More specifically, the added benefit is the humbling insight gained and his ability to share that insight in supporting, enhancing, and investing in our children, our people, and the future of our nation.

Raymond's first love is fitness training, he enjoys gardening, motorcycling, and writing. Writing is his way of exposing and countering the devastating systemic attacks on our children, in addition to arming them for generations to come.

Ase

Author and Book Website — www.rayjhead.com

Amazon Author Central — amazon.com/author/rjhead

Facebook @rayjhead Author — Raymond J Head

Instagram — rayjhead

www.ingramcontent.com/pod-product-compliance
Lightning Source LLC
Chambersburg PA
CBHW022250290526
45785CB00015B/501